S0-ECY-596

TECHNICAL MANUAL OF DEEP WHOLISTIC BODYWORK

Postural Integration

Jack W. Painter, Ph.D.

Also available by Jack Painter: DEEP BODYWORK AND PERSONAL DEVELOPMENT, Harmonizing Our Bodies, Emotions, and Thoughts (450 Hillside Avenue, Mill Valley, CA 94941, Tel. 415-383-4017).

Translations of the present volume are available in French, German, and Italian (write 450 Hillside). Translations of Deep Bodywork and Personal Development are available in French (Le Jour, Montreal), German (Koesel Verlag, Munich), Italian (Sugarco, Milano), Danish (Borgen Vorlag, Copenhagen), and Spanish (Ed. Pax Mexico, Mexico City).

Copyright 1987 by Jack Painter, 450 Hillside Avenue, Mill Valley, CA 94941, Tel. 415-383-4017. All rights reserved. Printed in U.S.A. No part of this book may be used or reproduced in any manner whatsoever without written permission except in the case of brief quotations embodied in critical articles and reviews. Shaded drawings in this volume are copyrighted by Chrisstine Fessler of Zurich. Copyrights to all other illustrations are held by Jack Painter.

Photographs by Margaret Boyles. Illustrations by Christine Fessler, Christopher Gouvea, Karin Lynch and Tim Tollfins.

TABLE OF CONTENTS

PART TWO

PREFACE

A few years ago the term "bodywork" had a rather narrow meaning. It usually referred to focused work on body tissues, using connective tissue manipulation, and massage. As the field of wholistic healing has rapidly expanded, a great variety of techniques are now used along with work on the body tissues. I always take the term "bodywork" to include work with thoughts and feelings and it would be, perhaps, more precise to use the term "bodymindwork." I use the term "deep bodywork" to distinguish between superficial massage and work with the basic bodymind structure. When working to transform bodymind, the layers of connective tissue, or myofascia, which envelop the musculature, are being freed and reorganized. Also I am concerned with "work," rather than "therapy," since to get therapy sometimes suggests that something is being done to someone. Truly effective and lasting deep bodywork depends on the active participation of the individuals seeking to change their lives.

In this manual I assume that the reader is either in training or has some experience in deep tissue work. I also assume that the reader has some knowledge of the fields of Bioenergetics or Reichian work, Gestalt work, acupressure massage, and movement awareness. If readers know little of these areas they can use this manual as a source book, consulting it as they gain enough knowledge to follow the discussions. There is, of course, a great deal of material which can be easily understood by the general reader. I refer the general reader, as well as the practitioner, to my introduction to deep bodywork, **Deep Bodywork and Personal Development, Harmonizing Our Bodies, Feelings, and Thoughts**. I have included several sections of this work in the present manual.

The first part of this manual sets the overall framework for understanding how to do deep bodywork. There is a discussion of the need for a unified, varied approach, of the structure of a session, and of how breath work and emotional work, movement awareness and soft energy regulation are all important in deep tissue work.

In the second part I have outlined each session in a ten session process. The discussion for each session is rather detailed, yet is not intended to explain every step involved in deep tissue work. This part of the manual can best be used in a training course where there is individual guidance.

Thanks to Christine Fessler, Christopher Gouve, and Karin Lynch, and Robert Mueller for their helpful drawings and illustrations. Also thanks to Andreas Vontobel for his encouragement in completing this manual.

READING LIST FOR STUDENTS OF DEEP BODYWORK

Alexander, M.: The Resurrection of the Body (Delta)
Barlow, W.: The Alexander Technique (Knopf)
Bandler, R. & Grinder, J.:   Frogs into Princes.
                           Trance Formations
Bean, O.: The Orgone and Me (Fawcett)
Boadella, D.: Wilhelm Reich, The Evolution of His Work (Dell)
Cailliet, R.: Pain Series (Davis)
Connelly, D.: Traditional Acupuncture (Ctr for Trad. Acupuncture)
Clemente, C.: Anatomy, Regional Atlas of Human Body (Lee & Febiger)
Feldenkrais, M.: Awareness Through Movement (Harper & Row)
Grof, S.:   Realms of the Human Unconscious (Viking)
Hammann, K.: "What Structural Integration is and Why It Works."
                     Osteopathic Physician, March 1972
Heckler, Richard Strozzi: The Anatomy of Change (Shambhala)
Janov, Arthur: Primal Scream
Johnson, D.: The Protean Body (Harper Colophon)
Dychtwald, K.: Bodymind (Jove)
Keleman,S.:   The Human Ground.
                  Sexuality, Self, and Survival.
Living Your Dying. (Lodestar)
Kelley, D.: New Techniques of Vision Improvement (Interscience)
Kendall, H & F: Muscles;Testing and Function (Williams & Wilkins)
Kurtz, R.: The Body Reveals (Harper & Row)
Lockhart, R.: Anatomy of the Human Body
Mann, E.: Orgone, Reich, and Eros (Simon & Schuster)
Melzack, R.: The Puzzle of Pain (Basic Books)
Painter,J.:   Different language editions of a similar manuscript:
            Deep Bodywork and Personal Development (Mill Valley)
            Le Massage en profondeur (Lejour;Interforum)
            Koerperarbeit und persoenliche Entwicklung (Koesel)
            Massagio in Profondita (Sugarco Sedizioni)
            Postural Integration (in Danish) (Copenhagen)
Perls, F.: Gestalt Therapy Verbatim.
Rolf, Ida: Rolfing (Harper and Row)
Schutz, W.:   Here Comes Everybody (Harper and Row)
Thompson, C.W.: Manual of Structural Kinesiology (mosely)
Todd, Mabel Elsworth: The Thinking Body (Dance Horizons)

PART I

THEORETICAL AND PRACTICAL PREPARATION
FOR DEEP BODYWORK

Chapter I

DEEP BODYWORK AND WHOLISTIC TRANSFORMATION

This manual is about how we can change ourselves and help others change themselves. It is about a step by step process through which we can release the chronic tensions and frustrations which we have accumulated since infancy and through which we can open ourselves, letting blossom the vibrantly healthy and fully alive self which lies dormant in all of us. In this process toward more freedom and happiness we have to deal with our resistance to change. It may seem that most of us want to change, that we want to be more relaxed, healthier, more alive. But here lies the basic problem of human transformation. Although we say we want a different kind of life -- and may even be involved in many projects for improving ourselves -- there is a part of us which stubbornly resists any fundamental redirecting of our lives.

This part of us, which refuses to let go, is our armor. We call it armor because it is that aspect of us which, being afraid of possible pain and confusion, hardens and desensitizes our bodies and keeps our feelings and thoughts in careful control. Our armor is all those well developed postures for dealing with life -- rigid neck, held in belly, fat, rubbery waist. It is all those guarded feelings -- covered up sadness, held back anger, paralyzing fear. It is those often unstated but controlling beliefs -- If I try I'll be successful; If I'm kind to you, you should be kind to me.

Reflect upon your own behavior. Notice the little tricks for getting through the day; how you get yourself going in the mornings, how you keep high by not indulging in negative thoughts, how you put your best foot forward when you want to impress people. A large part of this behavior becomes second nature to us, set in motion unconsciously, and functions well for us up to a point as it protects us from pain and confusion. However, these habits also limit us and in the due course of time form a rigid structure which then inhibits our spontaneity.

One of the main difficulties in changing ourselves is that this armor is largely unconscious but remains in control even as we try to modify a part of us. Each time we attempt to change our lives, we are, in fact, using our already developed (and unconscious) postures and attitudes to deal with our problems, For example, if you over-arch your lower back, creating severe backaches, you might try to find relief by doing yoga exercises. But you would probably concentrate on exercises which are easiest to execute and which at the moment feel good, such as arching your back even further into a fish or cobra position.

In the long run such postures will simply increase your body imbalance and create more pain. Here an unconscious attitude is driving you to find relief, but in a way which reinforces the old body position. Even if you are very disciplined and work with yoga positions which flatten your back, you will, through the attitude you carry throughout your body, simply transfer the
tension and imbalance to another part of your body. In flattening out your back, you may round your shoulders and overcontractthe muscles in your chest.

Or take another example. If you are very hard on the outside of your body, you may welcome very deep relaxing massage. You might, through frequent and thorough manipulation of your hard exterior, begin to soften -- soften, that is, on the outside. Another unconscious part of you doesn't really want to soften completely; that would be too exposing, too frightening. So much of this outer tension simply shifts to deeper, protective layers of muscle and tissue. You still have a restrictive, limiting armor, only now it has retreated deeper inside you.

The tensions of the body are clearly inseparable from one another, and are part of our overall posture and habits. Work on any part of the body which does not also release the whole structure, the habitual attitude behind our posture, is not transformation but simply a rearrangement of our problems.

Even when we go further and try to be more complete, dealing with the emotions and thoughts which are connected with our physical pains and imbalances, we encounter a similar subtle evasiveness in ourselves. Whenever I say that I am willing to explore every part of my body and deal with my thoughts and feelings, as well, I may actually be using an unconscious part of my armor. Here there can be a hidden, implicit message: "I try, but nothing ever works for me" -- a message which manipulates my body and mind even when I believe I am releasing both. In all our deliberate behavior there are such fundamental unconscious emotional and mental attitudes which have developed along with our physical postures and which govern our well intentioned efforts to improve our lives.

I have found in working with myself and with others that what we need is a way of dealing with the entire self, the unity of every part of our body, the outside together with the inside, the unity of our bodies with our minds. As we change old, rigid body postures, we need also to change the accompanying rigid feelings and thought processes; or if we release blocked emotions and ideas, we need to free the muscles and tissues for new, more flexible movements.

What I want to share with you in this manual is a type of "bodywork"-- that is, a method which works directly with the muscles, the positions, the postures, and movements of the body -- but a kind of bodywork which is not just work on these physical aspects of the self but which also is direct work with the emotional and mental attitudes expressed by these physical activities. I call this method or process "Postural Integration." In explaining Postural Integration to you I will be describing a specific process which I have developed, but I will also be describing any type of bodywork which respects the need for unitary, whole, self transformation.

If you are unfamiliar with bodywork as a way of working toward transformation of the whole person, you might be surprised, when visiting a session. There you might find a practitioner hovering over an individual, bearing down with hands, fingers, or elbows, while the person sighs, moans, or even screams and kicks. You might see the practitioner working very gently: rocking, cradling, and caressing the individual, encouraging deep breathing, or perhaps entering into a dialogue to clarify feelings and ideas. What sense could you make of all this? It could appear to be a cult, ritual, or even perversion.

But when we recognize that we resist change at both the level of body and level of mind, we can begin to understand the need for diverse, simultaneous strategies for transforming both. Postural Integration is a bodywork in which the practitioner uses fingers, fists, and elbows to grip, twist, and shift layers of tissue and to reorganize the muscular system. This process is not bodywork in the sense that the body is being treated separately from emotion and mind, but is bodywork only inasmuch as the body is a tangible, immediately available shape or form for body and mind.

When the body is changing, the mind is also changing, for they are simply different aspect of the same unity, different ways of focusing on the same experience. This means that in order for my deep work with tissues of the body to be effective -- not simply a rearrangement of my habitual armor -- it has to be coordinated with the accompanying emotions and ideas. Postural Integration, as a form of wholistic bodywork, is bodymind or mindbody work. The practitioner recognizes that in touching the body, either superficially or deeply, that there is also contact, simultaneously, with both feelings and thoughts, and that in encouraging their expression one is also encouraging physical change. (In Chapters III and IV we shall see that Reichian and Gestalt methods are important to bodymind change because they help bring out the hidden, controlling attitudes, and unleash the held back energy of unclaimed, armored thoughts and feelings).

The extraordinary power of Postural Integration lies in the willingness to work with the client on many levels at the same time. As I encounter the body with my hands, loosening the deep muscular tensions, I look into my client's eyes. And as I apply pressure, I ask that person to share through sound, movement, and words what is happening -- what is sensed, felt, and thought. By maintaining this contact, this open sharing, the practitioner can be flexible enough to change the emphasis of the work to meet the changing demands of the whole person. The practitioner and client together, now work with tissue, now with words, now with sounds -- all the time recognizing the physical, emotional, and cognitive unity of the process. My experience has been that when either the practitioner or client is holding back part of him or herself -- even as a part of the self to be dealt with at a later time -- the changes which do occur are partial, temporary, or even disorganizing. In Chapter II, in describing the basic structure of a session of deep bodywork, I will discuss in more detail this delicate interaction between the practitioner and client. Also in Chapter V, "Movement Awareness," I discuss the importance of both the practitioner and client becoming conscious of how to physically interact with movements which are guided by a meditative kind of bodymind consciousness.

I emphasize that healing transformation is simultaneous change, because I have noted that there is a tendency among some healers to treat body and mind as if they are objects which affect each other causally over a period time. There is a temptation to assume that if we work to restructure the body in a new physical form, we will eventually bring about healthier feelings and thoughts. And conversely if we can get emotionally and mentally balanced,the effect, it is thought, will be to release our physical stress.

There are some bodyworkers, for example, who seek to bring the sections of the body into balance in relation to the earth's gravitational field. Legs, pelvis, torso, and head are seen as the sections or blocks which because of stress shift out of efficient alignment. They assume that if the sections of the body find a careful and precise balance, that the emotions will also be harmoniously affected. The technical manipulations of these same practitioners are often subtle and masterly, yet in my experience their approach leaves aspects of the self out of realignment. For me, physical manipulations, which are not simultaneously part of emotional and cognitive change, result in superficial and temporary rearrangements of some of the parts, instead of a complete and instantaneous restructuring of the whole self. Some of these same practitioners treat the body as if it were an onion with layers which are to be peeled off layer by layer. But as I have explained in Chapter VII, "Working With Core and Shell," we need to work simultaneously with the inside and outside of bodymind or the result is only a rearrangement of our armor.

It is true that when the whole self, the entire bodymind, is free and centered, we are also in physical harmony with gravity, but we can never achieve this physical balance, unless our changes begin happening in every dimension of us at the same time. There is no way we can first find physical balance and subsequently catch up emotionally and mentally.

I have discovered that there is still another side to real transformation. It is not just that we change in every dimension of bodymind, both inside and outside of ourselves, we also, as we truly transform ourselves, find a center, a stable place or direction, in which our changes can happen with order and understanding. Deep bodywork can help us breakdown our old armor, the contractions dividing our heads, hearts, and desires. As our previous attitudes dissolve, we need to see that we can maintain our spontaneity by accepting the natural flow of each new attitude into the next. Here we are working with the subtle energy of the body, the delicate balance of a unified consciousness. In Chapter VI, "Fine Energy and the Five Elements," I set forth a variety of methods including acupressure points for helping us maintain our centers.

Chapter II

GETTING STARTED

Initial Contact, Bodyreading, And Outline Of A Session

SHARING EXPECTATIONS

When your clients arrive for the first session, they may be afraid of you and the unknown things that are about to happen. If you immediately ask them to take off their clothes and begin pointing out the tensions in their bodies, they will probably become more insecure and begin to feel like flawed objects. They will then be giving up responsibility for their changes and creating expectations which you cannot fulfill.

A suggested first step is to just sit together and talk about what you expect from each other. You might at this point explain how deep bodywork is a process which can be tried out. If it doesn't seem to be right for the person, one can drop out after a session or two. And it is a process with ever deepening consequences: if one gets three or four sessions, basic changes will have begun to happen which need to be worked through to completion. A clear understanding and commitment is needed from both of you. It should also be made clear at this point that there may be some pain, but that it can be releasing and relieving pain; and that there will be pleasure and joy as well. The PI process will be a period of transformation and they should take this into account during their everyday lives. Perhaps major decisions about employment, etc. can be postponed until the end of the process. Also athletes, dancers, and other very active individuals need to be aware that after some of the sessions, the changes in the body structure are incomplete and that overvigorous movement may create muscle strains, pulls, or cramps. The bodymind is changing and may not fully realize its new powers and limitations. Point out that the best kind of movement uses the whole body in flowing, effortless motions such as in free form dancing, swimming, and walking.

The next step, before any clothes are taken off, before a bodyreading, might be to sit facing one another making eye contact and breathing together. (You can kneel together on top of the table). Of course, this kind of contact may be too intimate for some beginning clients. During this initial contact, you may begin asking how they feel. Don't let them go into "war" stories about what has happened in their lives (these can be interminable, armor reinforcing tapes). Keep them in the present, taking responsibility for what's happening. "What are you feeling now?" Where is the feeling?" are good questions to get them started. Also don't let them talk about the big "it," that backache, that pain in the leg or neck which they are treating like some unwanted part of them. "It hurts" can be changed into a personal, claimed experience "I'm hurting here." Begin helping them take responsibility right at the outset. By getting them to express what's happening you also get them quickly into the process of change and to begin to see problems that may arise again during the course of the session. See Chapter III, "The Release and Expression of Feelings Through Gestalt Work."

BODYREADING

Perhaps at this point you have established enough rapport to begin a body reading. Have your clients take off just the amount of clothing they feel comfortable removing. Often after the tissue work is underway, they may cast aside more clothing to help your work. Again, don't begin by saying some part of them is tense or out of alignment. Ask what they feel. Get their participation.

1. Getting Into And Exploring Feelings. As they begin expressing what's happening, be sure, as mentioned above, to help them take responsibility for what they feel, by having them use "I". There are two general ways you can help them get further into expressing themselves. The first is to have them exaggerate a feeling or body position. For example, if they are angry and this anger involves tension running through the arms, you might ask them to increase the tension, to go into their anger more, to even play with sounds, e.g., growling. The second way is to explore feelings and positions. If they are collapsed in the chest, you might suggest that they really inflate the upper chest, hold the position, and get in touch with the feelings which they may be avoiding. Perhaps these individuals are weak and collapsed because they are afraid of being powerful, and they need to begin to experience and see this. You here have a chance to focus on the positive changes that can take place. You might share, "I see your legs getting stronger, and you finding a really comfortable, supporting center for yourself," or "I feel you're going to get longer, that your hips are going to be thinner, and that you will feel light and flexible." Such simple sharing can create a strong, positive support for change. Later in the sessions you may want to come back to the feelings and positions, which you have initially exaggerated or explored, noting that after the work of a session, they may be easier to express and complete.

2. Connecting The Whole Structure. Not only will your clients need help in expressing certain tensions and feelings more completely, they will also need to be helped in connecting isolated problems or symptoms to their overall structure. If for example, they say, "I'm tense all the time, here in my left shoulder," they may be unaware that this is related to a high right hip and collapsing left ankle. Or they may feel a knot in the diaphragm without realizing how connected it is to stiff, locked knees. This is happening emotionally too. When one feels constricted and tight around the heart, it may be difficult to see how a large, seductive pelvis may be robbing feelings from the chest.

3. Avoid Being Overly Analytical. It will probably not be helpful to talk to your clients about what type of structure they have, that is whether they are burdened, rigid, etc. Many people grab on to these designations and begin judging their behavior in terms of them. A study of types (burdened, rigid, top & bottom heavy, needy, ecto-, endo-, mesomorphic, etc.) may be helpful to you, however, as long as you keep this information in the background and allow yourself to accept what your client is expressing and to accept your own intuitions. The same is true of anatomical analyses. When you talk too technically and analytically about muscles or structural patterns, you may take your clients away from the experience of themselves. (For a discussion of how to use types and other information, while maintaining rapport with the client, see the last chapter, "Between You and Me, Sharing and Transforming Bodymind," of Jack's book *Deep Bodywork and Personal Development*..

4. Share. It is also appropriate for you to give your impressions to the client. For example, you might come right out and say, "I feel you have an awful lot of anger, which you could express; I would like to see that anger." When we give our impressions, we can check them out, that is ask whether they fit. And we can be ready to give our impressions up if they don't fit. Don't be afraid of projecting. Fear of imposing your trip on somebody else may itself be a projection.

5. Keep A Record. It will be helpful to take "before" pictures -- side, front, and back -- which you and your clients can compare with "after" pictures for any of these sessions, certainly after session 10. Be sure that you have a black background with evenly spaced white cross stripes and that you keep the camerathe same distance before and after. Also you may want to take some basic measurements: weight, height, size of chest and waist. Be sure these are exact, e.g., measure the chest with an inhalation or exhalation. These pictures and measurements will help your client be more interested and involved in the process and will also provide you with learning tools. You can later give this information to your trainer for evaluation.

Another way to help clients be more involved is to encourage them to keep a diary, write down dreams, draw their conceptions of themselves before and after sessions. A "Bodywork Journal" with basic questions, exercises, and orientation to the sessions is included in these notes. You may wish to expand this journal and make copies to give to your clients.

OUTLINE OF A SESSION

Each session will begin with some kind of initial contact, then a bodyreading in which the client participates. Now you are ready for the next steps: preparation, deep tissue reorganization, and final fine energy work.

PREPARATION

Before beginning deep tissue work, it is very important to prepare your clients for deep work. The tissue moves, and reorganizes, if the person is really ready to accept and assimilate the tissue changes you are encouraging. Two kinds of preparatory work are needed: establishing the flow of charging and discharging energy and the balance of fine energy.

1. Equalize Charge and Discharge. First, we need to help our clients equalize the energy they are taking in (charging) and the energy they are giving up (discharging). The key to this charging and discharging balance is the breath. In the release of armor we practitioners are working with the habitual ways in which the individual blocks and controls breathing. If our clients take in too much air, they build energy without fully expending what is accumulating. On the other hand, if they throw out their breath with an extended, contracting exhalation, and delay their need for incoming air, they literally overextend themselves. There is, for example, the aggressive, active male who keeps his chest puffed out, or the passive, listless female who collapses her chest and tightens her diaphragm.

2. Go Further Into The Disequilibrium. One way of releasing armor is to encourage the client to increase the energy disequilibrium even further. When a person is overcharged, I may encourage a still greater charge through deeper, more rapid inhalations, until the energy buildup finally has to surge into a discharge. On the other hand, when a person is undercharged, I may then encourage even more exhalation, until in exhaustion, a greater inhalation, automatically occurs and the persons recharges.

15

3. Explore The Neglected Aspect Of Breathing. Another way of releasing armor is take attention away from that part of the breathing cycle which is overworked and focus on the neglected part. If a client's exhalation is excessive, if there is too much discharge, I often help in softening and slowing down the exhalation, while supporting deeper inhalations especially in those areas of the chest, belly, or back which are neglected. Conversely, when the inhalation is too great, I shift attention from deep breathing to a larger exhalation, often encouraging exaggerated force and sound.

4. Be Both Provocative And Soft. Helping clients reach a level of charge and discharge where they can accept deep tissue work may involve vigorous stimulation or provocation of breathing, or subtle, gentle encouragement of breathing. This leads us to make a distinction between coarse and fine energy. When I work to change my general bodymind posture -- my sway back, my hysterical fear, my schizoid tendency to analyze everything -- I am focusing on "coarse" energy. Here I am concerned with large blocks of energy, with deeply ingrained habits, which set the basic directions of my life. On the other hand, I can stay within the limits of my general bodymind attitude, and without trying to change my sway back, fear, or overanalyzing, I can refine and improve the circulation of the patterns already present. I am in this case working with my "fine" energy.

Before I invite my clients to change the coarse, overall structure of their breathing, or any part of their bodymind, I need to help them to center themselves, to refine and organize their energy. And each time I stimulate an overall, coarse change in their structure, I need afterwards to help them rebalance their fine energy. During this first phase we may work provocatively with the breath, but generally we want to focus on a preparation of this fine energy so that gradually, deeper, coarser more fundamentally changes may take place as the session progresses further.

DEEP, COARSE WORK

Many students of bodywork initially have the idea that if they learn exactly where in the anatomical structure they can make a certain type of hand, finger, or elbow manipulation, they can, with some practice, master the complexities of deep tissue work. Actually no amount of observation, study, or practice -- although important -- can substitute for the need to make contact with an individual through an inner attitude. When I, as practitioner, begin with inner sensitivity, all my movements, all my contact with the other person, are both receptive and initiating -- receptive in that I allow my force to adjust to the resistance or openness of the individual, initiating in that I take the individual beyond the limits of his or her armor.

1. Interaction of Practitioner and Client. Consider what happens when I, the practitioner, or you, the individual with whom I'm working, make contact only externally or superficially. If I push against you with an outer effort alone, then I cannot easily regulate -- increase, diminish, change -- my force. You would feel my hands unresponsive to your inner needs and defend with your outside armor. Since my effort may be too fast, too deep, too hard, or just the opposite, too slow, etc., you would either become tense or totally passive in your extrinsic musculature. There is, then, no real contact, only an outer clash or compromise. This kind of outer contact, not real touching and caring, simply reinforces our armor. I am dumping on you my old feelings of power, while you are using my assault on your outside armor to reinforce old patterns of self defense.

16

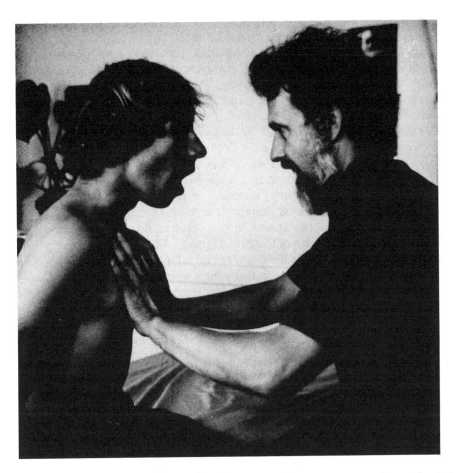

In wholistic bodywork the practitioner recognizes that in touching the body there is also contact with feelings and thoughts, and that one must encourage the espression of these in bringing about a physical change. The practitioner and client work together, now with tissue, now with sounds or words -- all the time recognizing the physical, emotional, and cognitive unity of the process.

Sometimes the practitioner and client begin their contact with careful intrinsic movements but then fail to follow through with complete external contact. If we begin together and I apply pressure so carefully that I adjust to every move I sense you making, I have only followed your needs without helping you discover new possibilities beyond your armor. Similarly if you submit inwardly to all my initiatives, you never discover your external power to give and interact.

In contrast to these incomplete attempts, full contact between you, the client, and me, the practitioner, is a special inner and outer reciprocity, a sharing in which we respect each other. Just as I move with and yet guide your inner and outer energy, you do not react, but dance with my pressure. This is a dance in which the dancer and the dance become one. It is a unifying movement of both of us, without action or reaction, only a simultaneity like the moves of opposing tai chi partners.

It may seem that the exchange cannot be equal. After all, you have come to me for help. How can you participate as an equal partner, if part of your armor is a defense against just such an exchange of energy, a resistance at some deep level to the possibility of your own self transformation? Even if I am centered and initiate my force from inside, and make sensitive, respectful contact with you, but you are afraid to surrender, how can the dance even begin?

For there to be a beginning in the healing process we need to recognize that both of us are incomplete in a paradoxical sense. You are resistant to change; that is the nature of armor. Yet you are willing to give up that armor when you are shown a possible path for change. I expect you to change. I want to help you overcome your blocks, yet I need to be very flexible, to change directions, if the direction I have suggested is not effective. In my role as healer, as Postural Integrator, I cannot completely accept your armored past. I work on the narrow border between imposing myself on you and accommodating myself to your old, armored games. The deep work with your tissue, blocked feelings and thoughts, elicits both pain and pleasure and is also a contact in which we feel resistance and release. If my force is too great or too painful for you, I will cut off the possibility of you beginning your own healing and transformation process. If my force is too weak or accommodating, I give up my power as healer.

Establishing and maintaining a delicately balanced exchange between the practitioner and individual calls for a variety of approaches and methods. Free, spontaneous breathing is essential to the cyclic balance of our energy, and when both the practitioner and client share and explore patterns of breathing in unison with each other, they are better able to sense the give and take needed in healing. All the integrating and fine tuning techniques help maintain this sensitive exchange.

2. Confrontation. This exchange allows for and encourages the direct expression of emotions arising from either practitioner or client. When I work with you, my role is to encourage you to explore the feelings that arise with the release of tensions you hold in your body, to confront and work through your unfinished business, and also to help you realize what you feel here and now about me. I need to give you my feelings of satisfaction, frustration, and sympathy. In this sharing it is not my job to remain emotionally   neutral or objective; but rather to give of myself and at the same time allow you the freedom not to live up to my expectations about how you can transform yourself.

The bodyworker and individual should both be free to project their needs on the other and to reject and accept the roles in which they are cast by each other. I am your parent; you are my child. I refuse to be your parent; you refuse to be my child. In the process of psychoanalysis the patient may slowly, over a period of perhaps months or years, transfer his or her parental needs upon the analyst, and thereafter gradually free him or herself from this transference. In the process of holistic bodywork (through direct and deep transformation of bodymind structures), we are continually and simultaneously both forming and breaking the transference. Of course, some period of time may also be needed for the integration and assimilation of this dual freedom into an individual's life.

3. Selective and Intuitive. In your tissue work respect the strategies we have outlined in Part Two of this manual for each of the ten sessions. Do not overwork. We have given you many more possibilities than you will need. Trust your intuition when it says to you, "Maybe I can work a little here and a little over there." In between strokes observe what has happened -- how the breathing is more connected, how the tissue stretches into a new area. Keep a charging and discharging breath going and work with the fine energy, brushing along the meridians as well as using acupressure points. Before ending a session be sure you have worked in enough areas to balance out the agonistic and antagonistic pulls of the myofascial system. For example, if you have worked on the belly and chest, work also on the back.

FINAL FINE ENERGY

This is the period in which we want to give space for clients to reorganize and balance the energy they have been releasing during the session. Always leave enough time for this fine tuning. What is especially important in all fine tuning is an attitude of not deliberately trying to change oneself. In fine tuning we have a general direction in which we want to move, a context in which we move comfortably, but we have no specific destination, no exact goal for our changes. Fine changes call for an open ended, spontaneous process of which we are mindful, attentive, meditative, but which we do not try to manipulate or control. I have found four areas of fine tuning especially useful in deep bodywork: breath regulation, energy distribution, movement awareness, and psychological redirection.

1. Breath and Charge-Discharge. Breathing is integrating when it flows freely through a cycle of charge and discharge, and recharge. In working to fine tune this breathing cycle, the practitioner helps the client sustain a meditative attitude through out a variety of breaths -- rapid, slow, even, uneven. By watching the breathing we realize that we can always return to a point where we can choose to follow, as our needs dictate, a given kind of breath without controlling it. We can become excited in our breathing, but see that we can and will return to a calmer rhythm. We can also play with expanding our breath along with large actions of the extrinsic, outside muscles and watch how we can quietly contract our breath with inner intrinsic movements. As we watch our expansion and contraction we flow with it.

2. Acupressure. Using the circular flow of the five elements, we can work toward a subtle balance of bodymind energy. Fine tuning with the five elements is not so much helping an individual find new energy or to get rid of excessive energy. It is rather the delicate distribution of energy throughout water, wood, fire, earth and metal. Using acupuncture points to regulate this flow requires a receptivity and consciousness. I look at my excessive fear and see that I can with the help of various points begin to allow this build up of water (fear) energy to spill over into wood (anger). I already have this energy. I need only allow it to follow its natural course. Consult the section in these notes on acupressure points and the five elements.

3. Movement. In several styles of working to make us more aware of our movements -- Alexander Technique, Feldenkrais Method, and Aston Patterning -- we find a recognition of the meditative and watchful but non interfering attitude. In the Alexander Technique we hold empty zen like images which we repeat but do try to execute. "Let the neck be free to let the head go forward and up, while the back lengthens and broadens," is an Alexander image which guides but does not follow the habitual goals we have built into our posture over the years. In Feldenkrais work the different parts of the body are given an opportunity to communicate with each other without the usual habitual commands. In stretching and exploring one side of my body I am already communicating, if my controlling consciousness does not interfere, with the other side of my body, and if my right arms moves more easily my left begins to recognize this and respond more freely as well. Or in Aston Patterning we are encouraged to find simple lines of symmetric movement, which we can explore by coordinating our whole body.

Perhaps these methods of movement awareness are such effective ways of fine tuning the bodymind because they give an opportunity to the nervous system to reorient itself. According to a wholistic interpretation, the gates in certain parts of the nervous system can be said to be set by previous painful experience, set by a protective armor which freezes the tissue in and around the muscles. As deep tissue is moved and freed, we relive and accept the event, gaining a new consciousness of the way we have previously set these gates. Now in fine tuning bodymind, we are able to begin resetting the gates for new kinds of experience which involve the whole nervous system.

In Chapter V, "Movement Awareness," you will find an outline of some basic movement awareness exercises, which when done in the spirit we have outlined above, can help your clients explore and accept the power of conscious movement throughout their bodies. These exercises can also help you in maintaining your own center while you work.

4. Affirmations. One way of redirecting our emotions and thoughts is to fine tune them with affirmations. Affirmations, when they remain open ended and are not attempts to manipulate ourselves, are ways for us to claim the power that has been released by the crumbling of our past armor. Whenever I repeat to myself, "I am opening myself to the love of other people," my affirmation is broad enough to give me a direction for change. But when I say "I can get Mary to love me," I am manipulating and armoring myself.

Affirmations are powerful means for fine tuning ourselves if they are not substitutes for dealing with the frustrations of life. An affirmation gives a context and direction for change, if we have already allowed our fear, rage, and sadness to be expressed and claim it as a part of us. But if our affirmations are simply means to overcome so called "negative" feelings, we have made ourselves unconscious for the sake of the false promise of an affirmation. "I am joyful and happy" is an appropriate affirmation only if we also allow ourselves, when the occasion arises, to fully experience our sadness.

It is possible that you may want to end a session by letting your client silently attend to whatever images may pass before their closed eyes. Place your clients such that their head falls back slightly and the arms are propped up at the elbows with the hands limp at the wrist. Instruct them not to move but simply follow the flow of images over the eyelids. It's o.k. if they fall into a sleep or semi sleep. This gives the nervous system an opportunity to process and rearrange the deluge of stimuli and reactions that have occurred during the session. Consider it as a period of rewiring or recircuiting.

Chapter III

THE RELEASE AND EXPRESSION OF FEELINGS
THROUGH GESTALT WORK

We have already seen that it is important simply to be there, to give your clients time and space to assimilate what is happening. Often this is enough, but if your clients are having difficulty sharing and expressing their feelings, you may need to understand something about the nature of their armor and how to help them come out of themselves.

RELEASING ARMOR

Armor is developed as a way of avoiding pain and dissatisfaction, but becomes the habitual means by which we unconsciously hold on to pain. For us to experience this armor is for us to begin to liberate ourselves from past attitudes and postures, but this is in no sense an avoidance or destruction of our unique personal histories. Encountering our armor is a distinct process in which we are freed from the past, and yet at the same time, make it part of us. In order to be free from our armor we not only have to contact it and acknowledge its role in our lives, we also have to contact it and acknowledge its role in our lives, we also have to claim it as a part of us. Helping our clients to allow this contact and to make this claim is our main job when encouraging the sharing and expression of feelings.

1. **Sense and Feel Incompleteness.** Often we so deaden ourselves that we become totally unconscious of our defenses and continually create an environment where we noeed not encounter any problems. Everything is carefully made safe and uneventful. The first condition for transformatio is to sense and feel our incompleteness, to be frustrated. During the release stage of Postural Integration, there comes a point at which clients begin to experience their resistance to change. Without this first step, no amount of tissue manipulation, deep breathing, guided movement, or spiritual and mental affirmation can bring about a significant and lasting release of bodymind armor. Encourage your clients to stay with what they are feeling, even if its uncomfortable, frustrating.

2. **Armor As Self Defense.** The second step in the experience of release is the acknowledgement or recognition that frustration, this sense of incompleteness, is the problem itself. So long as daddy, mommy, or society serve as the scapegoat for my problems, I will remain stuck, even if I am aware that I hae a problem. Equally, if it is "that back ache," or "those aching feet," which controls me, I have not yet acknowledged or recognized my armor for what it is, namely my defense against myself. The release I feel in letting go of my armor is not a mysterious event in which my burdens are relieved by some outside force. As the practitioner impinges on my body, I need to be willing to say "I'm resisting." With this recognition I may be feeling my struggle with myself, or I may simply be noting my resistance. Ask your client to notice their own avoidance and resistance.

3. **Self Acceptance.** Finally as a last step in the process of letting go of my armor, I need to claim my incompleteness, my pain and dissatisfaction as an important and welcome part of me. Now that I am responsible for creating my pain, I also accept it as a vital and valuable part of me. Here there is a seeming paradox: the moment I really accept my unwanted attitude, I become free from it. For example, when I accept my hatred for my father, the hate becomes complete, whole, and powerful, and I am

ready for other feelings. Now that I hate my father I can also more fully love him. The pain that emerges from deep tissue work is transformed. It is no longer raw pain but an accepted and claimed part of me which is no longer simply pain, but rather a release from an old hurt. I become free from my past by making it a part of me." Ask your clients to try out phrases such as "I am hurting myself", "I choose to make myself sick."

GESTALT AND ZEN VIEWS OF CONSCIOUSNESS

In order to better understand how old pain is transformed into a new free experience, we need a view of human consciousness which does not treat our bodies as objects to be analyzed and manipulated. In many of the classical western models of consciousness, consciousness is located in one place, "here," while the object is located "there," and we try to extend our awareness under controlled conditions by analyzing different parts of the object or event. According to this view, I see the pain in my lower back as a problem to be studied, as the effect of causes which I hope can eventually be understood and eliminated. But this separation of the pain from me is the problem. As noted earlier, so long as I deal with my pain as something foreign to me, I armor myself against the possibility of truly exploring the pain and being released from it.

Both the Zen and Gestalt views of consciousness make clear how the experience of being released is a process of claiming previously foreign parts of ourselves. When I fully contact, acknowledge, and claim a part of myself I am no longer just conscious of it as a separate object, I become the object. In Zen I totally blend with the object; I am both the observer and observed. And in Gestalt therapy, I illuminate the partly unconscious background of my experience by letting the unconscious part of me speak out.

As the practitioner encountered the well developed armor of my lower back, I felt the contact, I acknowledged my resistance to what lies deep inside me, and now finally I begin to claim my lower back by being there in it, talking from there to myself. "Jack, I'm huring; you've got to slow down the everyday pace and give me the attention I deserve." Even if this dialogue goes no further, I have already begun to release the unconscious defense which I have stored in my back. But not only can I release my armored parts, I can, through the now released parts, now comunicate with other aspects of myself which need to cooperate with each other, which need to try out new movements, feelings, and thoughts.

GESTALT TECHNIQUES FOR DEEP BODYWORK

Here are a few simple pointers to help you help your clients "gestalt" their feelings during sessions of deep work.

1. **Preparation.** Make adequate preparation by using the charging and discharging methods of breathing described in the next chapter, "Breathing and Energy Flow." If you make this preparation and maintain a high level of charge and discharge, even the most held back emotions will begin to surface.

2. **Start With the Here and Now.** The temptation is great to talk about the problem or to discuss what happened yesterday. Ask "What's going on right now." If they ask whether you mean in the body, or mind, or feelings, simply accept any of these. If they shake their head not knowing, ask them to repeat and exaggerate saying, "I don't know." In a gestalt session this first step usually takes a while and the first verbal expressions are often empty of much feelings. In bodywork, if there is no response we can continue with breath or tissue work, until the emotions begin to flow more readily.

3. **Deepen and Anchor the Flow of Feelings.** If your clients jump from one feeling to another or drift away into thoughts or fantasy, help them come back to what is happening. Ask what, or where are the feelings, and never "why." Exaggerating what's already happening is a good technique, when you begin slowly and gradually

with the movements, sounds, and words your clients are already using. You may want to continue your tissue work while suggesting that they continue to share what's coming up. If they become too active you will need to wait, before continuing the tissue work.

4. Direct Feelings Toward Persons. One way to anchor feelings is to make them specific. "I feel a lot of anger," can be turned into "I hate you." Don't be afraid to let feelings of resentment against you, the practitioner, come into the open. Encourage your clients to shout directly to you, "You're huring me," or "I hate you."

5. Encourage Self Acceptance. "It hurts," become "I'm huring." "They did it to me" becomes "I created this." The feeling of being a victim is, of course, a genuine feeling, and underlying it is also a level of self-victimization. Eventually all gestalt work begins with taking responsibilityu for all feelings. Even "My leg is cramping" is more completely claimed when it becomes "I am my leg and I'm cramping." We can do this with all the objects in our consciousness: "I am this room and I'm light and airy," etc. This process of identifying with the objects, ideas, feelings, and people around us is a powerful way we create our own unity and flow. As you penetrate tissue ask your clients to become that part of the body with which you are working.

6. Discover Background and Foreground. The unconscious parts of us are available if we just look at ourselves in a new way. We are like drawings which are tricks of the eye. If we allow our perception (experience) to change, the background can become noticed as the foreground. Help your clients notice that the parts of themselves with which they are most familiar are dependent on another unnoticed aspect of themselves. If they are very polite, no doubt they also have an enormous hidden rage. You might want to use some provocative Reichian techniques when you see an opportunity for the unexpressed side of y our clients to come to the fore.

7. Let Topdog and Underdog Interact. We all have a part of us which controls and another part which is controlled. If, for example, we usually play underdog, or victim, we can by a conscious choice shift our attitude and become the topdog which our underdog has been creating. Help your client get a dialogue going between the two parts. Use psychodramatic methods to support the weaker half. When the battle between the two becomes cooperation and sharing there may be a new insight, a momentary reshaping of the whole self, after reformation, ask one side what it really wants from the other and what it is willing to give. Also help explore the feeling that each side really needs the other.

8. Finished or Unfinished? At some point the interaction between topdog and underdog will have to take at least a temporary rest. Often it is enough that your clients feel both sides of themselves. There may be no resolution. But there can be a feeling that this is enough work for right now. Ask, "Are you finished for now?"

Chapter IV

BREATH AND ENERGY FLOW

Bioenergetic and Reichian Exercises

We have already seen in the "Outline of A Session" how it is important to work with the charge and discharge of breathing. Below I want to outline a number of exercises which you will find helpful in the ten sessions. In the later discussion (Part Two) of each session I will indicate which of these exercises may be especially helpful. If you use several at once, try to alternate the ones which bend the body backward with those that bend the body forward. Each can be used in either a provocative or soft way, and it is important for you to stay in touch with the ever- changing need for one or the other. Don't get stuck in using these exercises as only a way to charge or only a way to discharge. You may also use them not only as preparation for deep tissue work, but during the deep work to enhance the full release of emotions which are beginning to surface. You may also use some at the end of a session, along with affirmations, to reinforce new feelings and attitudes. I have explained these exercises in such a way that you can do them for yourself. You will, of course, eventually be assisting your clients.

Before turning to these exercises I want to discuss further the mechanism of breathing and to point out how in our work we are encouraging a special kind of spontaneous breath.

SPONTANEOUS BREATHING

The breath functions as a part of the whole bodymind and helps to establish a flexible balance by finding a level of recurring charge and discharge where our energy remains even and self-nourishing.

A complete cycle is not simply a repetitious building of energy followed by a discharge of energy , followed by another recharge. Nor is it an unbroken steady contraction, followed by steady expansion and then another contraction. An unarmored cycle of energy is made up of many smaller cycles, just as a liberating orgasm is a series of lesser, rising and falling orgasms. We see this in the rhythm of a free spontaneous breath.

Whenever I surrender and really let my breathing go, the rhythm is not merely in and out. As I inhale I quiver throughout the rib cage, and my whole breathing apparatus may even momentarily slow or stop the incoming air with subtle counter pressures, then continue with inhalation until I pause again. My inhalation is, then, an accumulation of small inhalations with some small countering exhalation-like movements. My exhalation is just the reverse: exhalations with partial momentary "inhalations."

This action is actually an interplay of the agonistic and antagonistic groups of muscles governing respiration. For example, the superior posterior serratus muscles in the upper back lift and open the rib cage during inspiration, while the inferior posterior serratus muscles in the lower back pull down and inward during exhalation. In alternating opposed movements, these muscles subtly check and free each other, eventually completely lifting up or pulling down the rib cage.

Not every inhalation or exhalation moves the total possible volume of air. The volume and depth of the breath varies continually with our physical, emotional, and mental demands, and the breath may change directions at any moment. An inhalation may, part way through, become an exhalation. The overall effect is a rippling, spontaneous rocking of the torso, which spreads up and downward through the whole body.

It is just this spontaneous, variable character of an unarmored breath which permits it to be complete. Each inhalation or exhalation, being free to pause or even reverse itself, is also free, under the right conditions, to fully expand or contract, to be a completely filled or empty breath. When we deliberately try to make breathing "complete," we create tension which prevents the variable streaming of energy necessary to the breath eventually completing its cycle. We then revert to using armored habits, and deal with ourselves as objects, instead of following the rhythm of our changing needs.

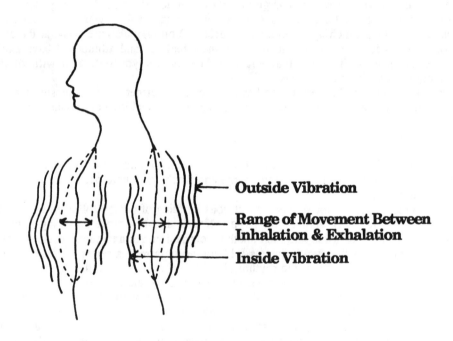

Outside Vibration

Range of Movement Between Inhalation & Exhalation

Inside Vibration

Breathing is a part of our whole bodymind. A spontaneous breath, that is, a breath which is full and free, helps us to establish a flexible center, a place from which our energy, our level of charge and discharge, remains even and self-nourishing. As we inhale, the breath quivers throughout the entire ribcage. We may even momentarily slow or stop incoming air with subtle counter pressure, then continue with inhalation until the next pause. An exhalation may also have these momentary, spontaneous pauses. The overall effect is an inner and outer vibration, which gently rocks the torso, and spreads throughout the body and mind.

The capacity to be flexible in every aspect of bodymind calls for a sustained and equal level of both charge and discharge. The breath now can be charging, or now discharging, but it equalizes itself. In contrast with the initial release stage of work, in which we exaggerate or support over and under-accentuated parts of the breathing cycle, during the integrating stage of Postural Integration, I help clients explore their capacity for variety and duration in breathing. I encourage them to experiment with charging by alternating between rapid and slow, shallow and deep, excited and calm breaths. Practitioners need to work with such sensitivity to the movement of their clients' breathing that their own bodies and breathing rhythms synchronize with even the slightest change in the direction of the breath. Frequently I take my clients through cycles of charge and discharge where a single charge can be a long series of ever increasing inhalations, finally reaching a plateau, but the charge does not become excessive because it is always balanced with some discharge. I help them gradually descend from this plateau by focusing on a series of increasing exhalations, until charge and discharge are balanced at a lower level.

EXERCISES FOR OVERALL ENERGY FLOW

1. The Bow. The feet are spread (not too wide or too narrow). The toes are turned inward. The whole body is arched upward and backward from the ankles to the top of head. Be careful not to concentrate too much arch in the small of the back or in the back of the neck. The fists rest on the back of the hips with the elbows pointed backward. Adjust the knees, flexing or extending them slowly until you find the point at which your body begins to vibrate. You may find that only one part of your body, the thighs or belly, for example, will vibrate, indicating that other unmoving parts are heavily armored. You may need to stay in this position until, after having breathed for some time, there is adequate charge and discharge for the vibration to begin. Maintaining the position, keep on deep breathing for at least five minutes. Remember that if you need more discharge, focus on the exhalation, along with perhaps a crisp "ha" sound, and if you need charging, focus on the inhale, with a softer exhale. Work with both feelings of being grounded and uplifted.

2. Between Heaven and Earth. Same as Bow, except the arms are extended above the head, the elbows passing along a line even with the ear.

3. Forward, Surrendering Bend. Legs are the same as in the Bow. Bend forward at the waist until the hands touch the floor. Don't use the hands for support. Sometimes shifting the weight forward onto the balls of the feet will help create more vibration. Explore feelings of being grounded while letting go.

4. Wood Chopper. Combines elements of Between Heaven Earth and the Forward Surrendering Bend. From Between Heaven And Earth position swing forward giving an exhale and relaxing into swinging of arms between the legs. Swing back up with an inhale until arms and head are back. Be careful not to over arch the back or neck. Begin slowly until you find a smooth back and forth swinging rhythm. In this exercise we are combing discharge and charge. You may, of course, focus more on one or the other.

PANTING

1. High Chest Pant. Hold the belly in, forcing the air into the upper chest. Pant, beginning slowly and gradually increasing the rhythm. Keep the chest high without breathing in the diaphragm.

2. Belly and Waist Pant. While on back, prop the pelvis up high with the elbows. Breathe only into the belly, letting it balloon out on the inhalation. Slow down the panting, if it becomes confused. A vigorous shout on the exhale can help.

27

NEEDINESS, COMMITMENT, AND SURRENDER

1. Picking Fruit. Reach with one arm toward a bunch of imaginary fruits which are almost out of reach. If standing, go up on the toes and stretch the side of the body. If on the table sit up on the hip or knee. Inhale with the reach. Explore feelings of going for it, of commitment.

2. The Crab. Lie on your back. On the exhale, reach with both arms, letting the head drop back and shoulders go forward (upward). At the same time (with the exhale) the legs, which are propped up and bent at the knees, fall outward until the legs are spread. On the inhale bring the knees together and lower the arms to the sides. On the exhale you can explore "I want you," or "Come to me." The practitioner can stimulate the groin area by slightly pinching with the thumbs and forefingers around the gracilis.

3. The Jelly Fish. While you are on your back, keep your arms extended above, shoulders following and head falling back. The knees are pulled up toward the head, so that the belly stays slightly contracted. Make small circles with your knees until a vibration sweeps through the whole torso and the circles become more confused.

ANGER

1. Lebensraum (Give Me Space). With fists clenched, vigorously swing the elbows alternately from side to side, exhaling with each swing. Unleash your pent up anger with shouting and growling.

2. Marching. While lying on the back, begin mechanically to stamp alternately with your feet and pound alternately with your fists. You can count, "1,2,3,4." Exhale with each number. Gradually increase the tempo. As your "marching" becomes more vigorous, let yourself fly into a wild, crazy rage. The practitioner can give encouragement by deep massage of the masseter and temporalis. Be sure there are enough pillows and mattresses to protect you.

3. The Barking Dog. While on your hands and knees, inhale, tucking your chin and head in, and curling your pelvis toward your nose. As you exhale, throw your head up and out and arch your back at the same time, making a loud "whoof." The practitioner can slap along the back and buttocks, or grab the trapezius and hamstrings to encourage the release. The back and anus hold a lot of held back anger against parents or authority. Try screaming "Mommy" or "Daddy."

4. Grand Slam. This can be done with a tennis racket or with the fists. From a kneeling position, swing back over the head and slam down into the pillow, while exhaling and crying out. Again, shouting out the name of someone can be effective.

5. Snap Kick. While on back kick with one leg into the air, shouting and exhaling. Let this kick snap through the whole body beginning at the ankles and reverberating all the way to the neck and head. When done forcefully, the whole body is launched into the air sideways. It is good to direct this anger toward a specific individual.

6. Pelvic Drop. Lift the pelvis with an inhalation. Drop the pelvis onto a soft mattress or pillow and shout "no." Try lifting higher each time and shouting louder.

POWER AND ASSERTIVENESS

1. The Ape. Inhale very deeply. With the chest inflated, beat out the exhalations by raping on the chest and roaring. Reinforce the feeling that it's o.k. to be powerful, to be in control.

28

2. Filling Up. Take a series of short inhalations without exhaling. With each inhalation expand the chest further. Explore the feeling of being expanded.

3. The Bear. Bend over at the waist, head and arms hanging free. Walk with stiff legs, letting the torso swing forward with each exhalation and grunt. Move without advancing, while pushing against the wall or another person.

4. The Splattering Snow Flake (The Andreas Vontobel Special). Stick out your belly and collide with someone else's belly, exhaling and shouting as you make contact. Try the same but meet belly to belly in midair. Explore the feeling of not only being powerful but making contact with someone else who is also powerful.

5. Spread Eagle. While lying on the back, let bent knees flop and extend arms outward (not upward as in crab) and with a vigorous exhale shout "yes."

FEAR

1. Shock Mime. Practitioner hovers over the client. Both hold eyes and mouths wide open with hands spread open alongside the head. Maintain this expression, while practitioner draws eyes closer and closer. Rapid breathing and shouting can also be explored.

2. Baby Curl. Curl up in an embryonic position. Alternately tighten and relax the whole body.

3. Choking. Hold the throat, cutting off just enough air to provoke coughing. Use either the whole hand around the throat or press the thumb or finger directly on the middle of the trachea, just below the adams apple. When coughing begins, beat gently on chest and back to encourage a full release. Explore the fantasy of the worst possible thing that could happen. If the feeling of dying comes up, ask what it feels like to die, and ask "O.k. now that you're dead what do you feel."

SADNESS

1. Chest Depression. The practitioner presses down on the chest with each exhalation. Vibrate the hands as you press and gradually, with each exhalation, press further until the exhalation is more complete and blocked feelings begin to   emerge. Also you can keep your hands on the chest until the client begins coughing or crying. Another way to evoke deep sadness is to put the weight of your body (chest) on the client's chest and wait, gradually giving more and more of your weight.

2. Inner Nose. Wet the little finger and slowly insert in the nostril. Gradually open the different conchi (cartilaginous passages). As you go deeper the eyes will begin to water. After removing the little finger, explore any sad feelings.

3. Half closed eyes. Close the eyes slowly half way. Maintain this half way position, just at the point where the eyes quiver. This may prompt tears.

DISGUST

1. Gag. Place your first finger deep into throat to activate gagging. Keep the finger there just long enough to start the reflex. Reinsert the finger briefly to keep the reflex going. When possible don't stop to clean the mouth with tissues until after one has really gotten fully into a series of gags. Direct the feelings of disgust toward specific individuals. This vibration may also turn into a feeling of relief and sadness.

2. Blahs. Stick the tongue out as far as possible and shout "blah" from the gut. Each time increase the force of the exhale until one is doubling over in mild spasms, perhaps with coughing and choking.

CENTERING

1. Eye Focus. The practitioner uses a pen light, pencil, or finger to direct the eyes in circles, squares, figure eights, and other irregular patterns. This is done slowly in the beginning and then unpredictably. Also try moving from far away to a point in the center of and close to the eyes, then moving quickly further away.

2. Whammy. Suddenly without warning the practitioner slaps the hands together in front of the face of the client and asks "What are you feeling now."

SENSUALITY

1. Roof Tickle. Rub the palette of the mouth with your finger. Often the person shivers and you can gently stroke the whole length of the body.

2. Sucking. Suck your thumb and hold your genitals at the same time. Explore simultaneously neediness and satisfaction.

3. Biting. Bite the heel of your hand without drawing blood. Bite a towel and hold on while its being tugged. Biting is not necessarily an expression of anger. It may be a playful way of making intimate contact.

4. Stand Me Up. Slightly rub and pinch the nipple tips until they become erect. Combine this with gentle rubbing of the whole body.

5. Sexual Surrender. With the legs open, massage the groin area with thumb and fingers around the gracilis. This can be pleasurable.

6. Rock and Roll. While on the back with knees bent, gently curl the pelvis toward the nose. Inhale as you curl up. Don't arch the back on the exhale. Gradually increase the rate of the rock until you are panting, rocking, and vibrating. Have a fantasy of something (someone?) you really want. Let it be alright to be excited.

7. Tickle. Enjoy being tickled all over. If you want to go further, explore the anger and helpless that may be underneath by being tickled to the point of rage or desperation. Tickle the bottom of the feet or the armpits.

8. Face Stimulation. Rub, gently pinch, and shake the face. Let this be playful contact, breaking all the taboos about being careful not to be too intimate with the face. Try out playful sounds at the same time.

9. Bottom Rub. Massage, roll, and shake the bottom. Alternately tighten the buttocks. Lift the bottom in the air and spread the cheeks. Stay in touch with your fear and anger and dare to surrender to your sensuality.

Chapter V

MOVEMENT AWARENESS

We saw in the "Outline of a Session" that clients play an active role in interacting with the practitioner. Not only must they be willing to actively charge and discharge their energies and take responsibility for releasing blocked feelings and attitudes, they need also to carefully move their bodies to interact with the practitioners pressure and to explore their new flexibility. And as the practitioner gives his energy he needs to maintain his own balance and center. Both the practitioner and client need to understand how to move with awareness and freedom.

We have also seen that a meditative, non-efforting consciousness is important to easy, free movement. If I am trying to accomplish a specific goal my body prepares itself by contracting according to habitual patterns. If I want to get up and shut the door, the muscles of my neck and back begin to tighten, as they always have when I have stood up. In breaking free of these habits I need to let myself unify with my environment, so that I am extended throughout my space. I am in a sense the room and the door. If then I move in a direction, rather than toward a specific goal, such as closing the door, I simply expand part of me toward the door. I spontaneously move in wave like movements in that direction and in the process my door gets shut. My directives are not specific goal-oriented commands, rather they are empty, zen like images, e.g., "I am moving upward; I float this way: I contract back in this direction."

In helping clients find this kind of spontaneous movement you can give them meditative images. You can also gently guide their bodies. Placing your hands on the shoulders or back, you simply wait for them to follow the spontaneous movement of your hands in a given direction. This can be especially helpful at the end of a session, after the deep tissues have softened and the emotions and thoughts are flowing more freely.

During the deep work itself, you can invite your clients to slowly move into your pressure, to follow a direction of movement which leads to those areas which need and want to be touched and released. But if they try too hard they will be using their armored habits to deal with stiffness and pain in the old defensive ways they have always used. Finding the place, the pressure, the attitude which has been largely unconscious is then part of our goal. I might say when working with someone, "It's o.k. for you to scream and kick like this when you feel pain, and it is important for you to move and express yourself in ways that you have been avoiding; try surrendering and accepting the pain and moving more gently."

All free, spontaneous movement is only "in a direction" and never toward a specific goal. The following exercises, although they have been written as a set of instruction should be taken in the spirit of exploration, without effort.

These exercises begin at the feet and proceed step by step to the neck and head. Take at least an hour in the beginning to practice these exercises. After you have mastered them, you can run through them in ten minutes. You can use them in three ways: 1) as movements which your clients can use to interact with your deep tissue work, 2) as movements which they can explore after a session to enhance their new flexibility, 3) as a complete set of centering exercises which they can use in between sessions and for permanent maintenance, 4) as a set of exercises and principles which you can use while doing deep tissue work in order to stay centered.

PRELIMINARY ORIENTATION FOR MOVEMENT

1. **Parallel Lines.** Imagine the body as organized along two parallel lines. When the legs are turned in or out or if they are spread too wide or too narrow, the body cannot move efficiently along these straight ahead rails.

2. Right Angle Axes. Imagine that the body functions by means of a series of axes at right angles to these parallel lines. These axes pass through the joints at the toes, ankles, knees, pelvis, mid-thorax, and head. If these axes are tilted away from right angles, the body alignment moves from side to side.

3. Stacked Blocks. Imagine a vertical line which passes through the ankle, pelvis, mid-lateral thorax, and ear. If this line is tilted forward or backward, the segments of the body can no longer stack one on top of the other. The image of a dragon tail can help bring the pelvis from a swayed position into easy alignment. The image of the thorax opening evenly outward like an umbrella helps make the cage rounder and more balanced. The image of a string lifting from the crown of the head allows a chin which is lifted too high to drop down.

4. Shaking Tree. Imagine that this whole structure is not static, but vibrates in waves and pulsations with the line of balance always changing.

5. Tide. Imagine that the structure expands and contracts in spontaneous and ever-changing rhythms.

EXERCISES FOR FEET

(From sitting position, knees up and in alignment). These instructions are reminders for students who have already been guided through the exercises and are not an independent guide.

1. Toe Wake Up. Feet are flat on floor. Toes moving together, up and down. (Remember all these exercises are along the parallel lines and axes of the body).

2. Tip Toe. Toes up, ankles up, ankles down, toes down.

3. Toe Scrunch. Pull toes under, then ankle up, toes up, ankles down, toes down.

ROTATION OF LEGS

(From sitting position, legs extended, knees locked).

1. Achilles Tendon Stretch. Ankles up, rotate legs out.

2. Tip-toes. (Toes up, arched foot). Rotate leg out.

3. Ballerina Toes. Rotate, tracing semi-sphere.

ANKLE AND KNEE COORDINATION

(Sitting position, legs extended).

1. Automatic Flex. Bend one knee, move the knee by moving the foot up, rolling on calcaneous. Do not use the hamstrings or quadriceps. Place your hands around the thighs to make sure.

2. Super Knee Bend. With knee already bent, begin movement of knee by moving foot as above. Continue flexing the lower leg with achilles tendon stretched until heel reaches buttocks.

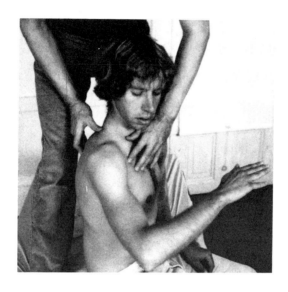

Deep bodywork can help a person establish an easy balance between different muscle groups. Often when we move an arm, we unconsciously overstretch muscles in the middle of the back, (the lower rhomboids), which help to hold the scapulae and shoulders in place. When this happens the opposing muscles on the front of the body (e.g., pectoralis minor) are overcontracted, and as the arm moves forward, so does the shoulder. Here the practitioner is working simultaneously on the rhomboids in the back and the pectoralis minor in front, encouraging the client to move his arm from the elbow, while keeping the shoulder stable.

PELVIS

(Lying on back, knees up, feet on parallel lines, chin in, shoulders down).

1. Pelvic Curl. Curl pelvis, using psoas. (See notes on intrinsic and extrinsic muscles).

2. Pelvic Curl With Lift. At the end of the curl continue until the pelvis is slightly lifted. Come back down one vertebra at a time.

3. Pelvic breath. Inhale with pelvis curl. Take air all the way to collar bone and up the throat to the third eye. Exhale down the spine. Imagine the air going out your tail bone and feel a slight automatic rock in the pelvis. (See instructions for this exercise in Chapter V of Deep Bodywork and Personal Development).

COORDINATING PELVIS, BACK, AND SHOULDERS

1. The Monkey. Squat with back flat. Spine is slightly rounded forward. Back of neck is flat. Shoulders are back arms hang free.

2. Monkey With Shoulder Pull. From the monkey, hold both arms behind the back, pull shoulders down and back using lower, not upper rhomboids.

COORDINATING SHOULDERS, NECK, AND ARMS

(On back, knees up, arms extended, elbows locked, thumbs down, palms toward ears).

1. Crucifix. Bring arms together, in front of chin. Return down to floor. Shoulders are kept in place by rhomboids. Notice the unevenness of arm movements: how one arm may want to be higher or lower than the other. Explore the angles and areas through which you do not want to move.

2. After a quarter rotation of the arms, the palms will be up. Repeat #1.

3. After a quarter rotation, the thumbs will be up. Repeat.

4. After a quarter rotation, the palms will be down. Repeat.

5. Reach to Heaven. (On back, knees up, arms down at sides, palms down, and elbows locked). Bring arms up, along parallel lines, all the way over the head until the backs of the hands touch or almost touch the floor. Keep the shoulders down by using the lower rhomboids. Now rotate the hands until the palms are down as you sweep along the floor and reach the original, beginning position of the arms.

INTEGRATION

1. Spinal Roll. (Sitting on the edge of a chair or on knees). Rock to find a point of balance. Drop the neck forward, bending the uppermost cervical vertebrae, the thoracic and lumbar vertebrae. Reverse the sequence and let the neck finally go back into position. Repeat 10 or 15 times until the vertebrae move freely and independently.

2. Side Stretch. (On back with knees bent; hands are together over the head). Cross right leg over left. Shoulders stay down. Swing legs to the right at least 20 times. Keep the hands together and in position even as legs flop to side. Reverse by putting left leg over right and letting legs fall to the left.

3. Pelvic and Third Eye Breath. (On back with knees bent). Do pelvic curl as above and imagine that a string gently pulls the anus and genitals upward to the third eye with each inhalation and let the string then relax on the exhalation when the pelvis drops. This is a very subtle, easy movement.

4. Pelvic Curl Coordinated With Legs and Arms. (On back with knees bent, arms bent, lying against floor with palms up). While doing pelvic curl, stretch the achilles tendon. At the same time pull the elbows down along the floor. Back and neck stay flat, knees stay on parallel lines.

Chapter VI

WORKING WITH THE CORE AND SHELL

In working with our clients we need to be aware that the body (and mind) defenses form protective layers which need to dissolved gradually but not necessarily layer by layer. First let us look at how armor divides itself into an outside and inside part, and then, at the general strategies for working with this armor.

DEVELOPMENT OF CORE AND SHELL

Growing up is a process of developing responses, many of which we turn into rigid habits for protecting us against pain, but which also restrict our experience and spontaneity. The earliest of these habits form the core of resistance. During the trauma we experience at the beginning of life -- during the moment of conception, while moving along the fallopian tubes, and when implanting and gestating in the uterus -- that early in our existence we are already establishing patterns for handling the world and protecting ourselves. We reinforce this developing, protective core as we are forced to cope with the shock of birth, and to then struggle through the oral, anal, and genital phases of our infantile growth. By the age of three or four years, we have almost fully developed our characteristic postures, our ways of avoiding pain and unwanted change.

The rest of our lives is usually a reinforcement of this core, years of similarly accumulated protective responses. But we make our armor even more complicated by creating more protection: a veneer placed around this core. For although the core is the most resistant part of us, it is also the most vulnerable to intense pain. The shell may allow us to take some risks. If we get hurt there, it is superficial, and we are still protected at the deeper level.

We maintain this basic division between core and shell in many forms. Sometimes, the body itself can reveal a hard exterior of well developed, extrinsic muscles (for locomotion), covering a center of weak, intrinsic muscles (for balance). Consider as an example the muscle-bound athlete, who has temporary strength but no grace. Conversely, the outside can be a soft physical buffer around a tight but passive center. Look at the "delicate" feminine type woman who is "hard as nails" under the surface. This separation into outside shell and inside core also happens at the emotional and cognitive levels. Our everyday social feelings may be flat and controlled, yet cover deeper explosive emotions. Or if we are gregarious, we may, nonetheless, hold back inner feelings of doubt and fear.

FLUIDITY OF INSIDES AND OUTSIDES

The alternative to this armored splitting of ourselves into a core and shell is to move, to feel, to think with our whole being, letting what is happening in our outside life be what is happening in our inside life. When we are most alive, that is, fully responsive to our environment, as well as active in it, our energy is not limited to surface reactions or to inner initiatives. Fear, anger, joy, sympathy, and grief move freely through us, from the outward contact with the people around us, pouring right into our deeper feelings of empathy and sharing. At the same time, those emotions can begin inside us and without repression flow outward toward others. Thus when we are fully alive, the core and shell both disintegrate, and our energy moves easily from outside to inside and from inside ot outside.

Reaction and action are different view of the same event. My reaction to you is a mode of my action toward you. When you touch me, my response is my active acceptance or rejection of you. My inside and outside energetically function together as aspects of my single unified reality. This unity can be felt in the body tissue. When there is unity, there is balance between the larger extrinsic muscles (which give power to our movement) and the deeper intrinsic muscles (which give subtle direction and stability). The unarmored, active and receptive individual has a consistent, soft yet firm tone from the skin inward to the deepest structures.

If we become conscious of the overdevelopment of the outside of ourselves, of the hard protective shell we have created, we might try to soften this defense by working gradually from the outside toward the core. One of the most frequently used strategies in deep bodywork is to work from the shell to the core. In this work the body is considered to be layered like an onion, and in order to affect and reach the inside layers, the outside has to be peeled away.

We can understand this approach to the body better, if we look, for a moment, at the nature and arrangement of the tissue being manipulated. The muscles of the body are wrapped in envelopes, consisting of a pliable tissue called fascia. This material organizes and guides our muscles by forming a system made of layers of tissue. On the outside of the body we have a large, all encompassing layer, which like a big shopping bag holds everything together. As we go deeper we find individual sheaths for each muscle. As we develop rigid physical and emotional patterns of behavior this system of fascia becomes less flexible, restricting our movements and overall bodymind attitude. The strategy in this kind of work (from outside toward inside) is to soften and reorganize those parts of the fascial system which have become hard and stuck, and this, in turn, it is thought, gives mobility and balance to the muscles held in the fascia.

I have found that if we begin working with the outside of ourselves. in the belief that we can affect and make more available our insides, we overlook how our armor subtly shifts its defenses. The tension that we release superficially may simply move toward a deeper more protected place. It is, of course, important to respect the rate at which a person undergoes and assimilates change, and often in my work I focus on the outside superficial planes of fascia, and then gradually go deeper. Yet I have found that when real transformation occurs, it is not only the outside that is changed. The inside is also simultaneously undergoing corresponding changes.

As I begin working with superficial layers of tissue, I am coordinating this work with the individual movement of intrinsic muscles, such as gentle rocking of the pelvis or short, slight movements of the spine. Also as I work with the extrinsic musculature, as well as the outer feelings and attitudes, I may, for example, work simultaneously inside the mouth, which holds some of the deepest structures, emotions, and attitudes of the body. Rather than viewing the body, the bodymind, as a many layered onion, I see it as a vibrant plastic mass, less viscous in some places than others, and composed of the same interflowing stuff from outside to inside and from inside to outside. Thus when touched at any level or depth, it instantaneously responds, reshaping itself in every other dimension and part.

TECHNIQUES LOOSENING AND REORGANIZING FASCIA

Although we are always working with all the layers of fascia simultaneously, we do in the beginning concentrate on the superficial, next the intermediate, and finally the deep. My use of these three layers does not correspond to any one system of anatomical classification but is a mixture of classifications taken from German, French, English texts. (See A. Forster, Ueber die morphologische Bedeutung des Wangenfettpfropfes; A. Richet, Traite pratique d'anatomie medico-chirurgicale; E. Singer Fasciae of the Human Body and Their Relations to the Organs They Develop; and B.B. Gallaudet, The Planes of Fascia). What I call "superficial" comprises both the fatty and denser subcutaneous layers. What I call "intermediate" is referred to in some texts as the "superficial subserous fascia," and what I call "deep" as the "deep subserous fascia."

In working with fascia we are interested both in softening and reorganizing it. Sheets of fascia have a tendency to thicken and adhere to surrounding tissues. An important part of our work is to separate these sheets of fascia such that muscle fiber can soften and function more freely. In the separating and softening process we need to pay attention to the depth of our strokes. In the following diagrams you will see that depth is controlled by the angle at which we apply force with fingers, fists, etc. Depth is also to a certain extent controlled by the amount of force we use. (But this is not nearly as important as beginning students sometimes think).

We also need to encourage the coordination of different parts of the fascial system. In superficial work we are working with flat broad strokes toward a spreading of the outer body envelope, a general, spacious, fluffing out of the whole subcutaneous layer. In intermediate work we go slightly deeper with shorter strokes and begin touching and opening individual myofascial envelopes, the wrappings around each muscle. In deep work we are going in between and under envelopes. Now our strokes are very slow and short.

During the final phase of work, session 8, 9, 10, we use a special type of stroke which is almost as broad as superficial work (we want to encourage major sections of fascia to shift with each other), but it is also deep enough to move all three layers of fascia (which are now soft and more malleable).

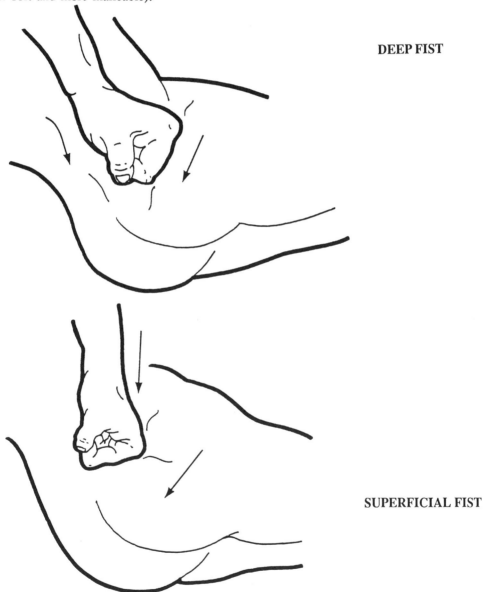

DEEP FIST

SUPERFICIAL FIST

A superficial stroke uses a slightly open fist over a broad area, while a deep stroke is shorter, firmer, and more specific.

**SECOND AND THIRD FINGERS
REINFORCING FIRST FINGER**

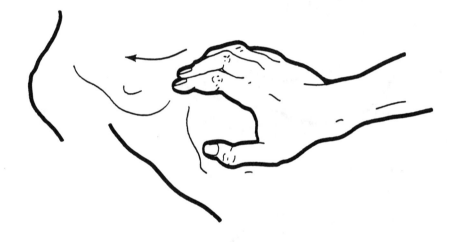

As illustrated this stroke is superficial, but it can also be made deep. In either case it is important that the fingers be kept arched and not allowed to buck inward.

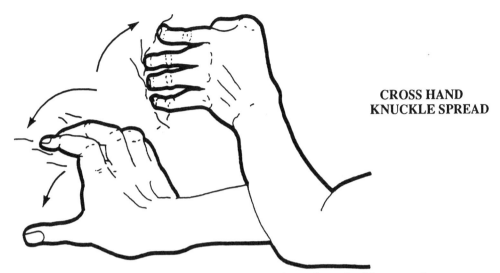

CROSS HAND KNUCKLE SPREAD

When this stroke is used with the hands at a wide angle and with outward movement, it spreads superficial fascia over a fairly wide area; it is used extensively in sessions one and two. If the angle were more acute, more force applied, and the storke shortened, it would then be appropriate for the intermediate and deep work of sessions 3, or 4 through 7.

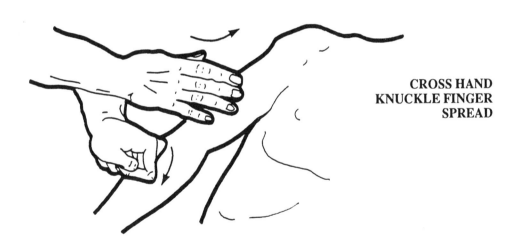

CROSS HAND KNUCKLE FINGER SPREAD

This stroke is also a superficial stroke, appropriate for the beginning sessions. When, however, either the knuckles or the hand is used to anchor the tissue and one hand penetrated more directly over a shorter distance, then the stroke becomes deep and begins separating tissue rather than spreading it, and would consequently be used only after the superficial work is complete.

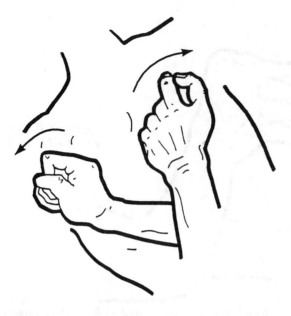

**CROSS HAND
KNUCKLE SPREAD**

The same is true for this position as for the Cross Hand Finger Spread on the previous page. Notice that in both cases there is not just an outward movement, but also a spinning motion which helps hook and hold the tissue being spread or separated. This hooking of tissue is essential to all connective tissue work.

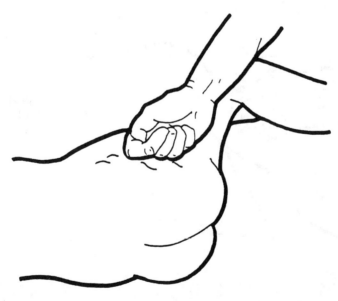

**FIRST KNUCKLE
REINFORCED WITH
THUMB**

This is a basic hand position, which can be used in either a superficial, intermediate, or deep stroke.

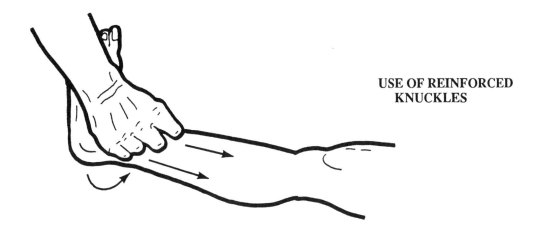

USE OF REINFORCED KNUCKLES

This stroke can be superficial, intermediate, or deep, although reinforcing the first knuckle with a second helps in deep work. In order to get good tissue separation or spreading, add a twisting motion.

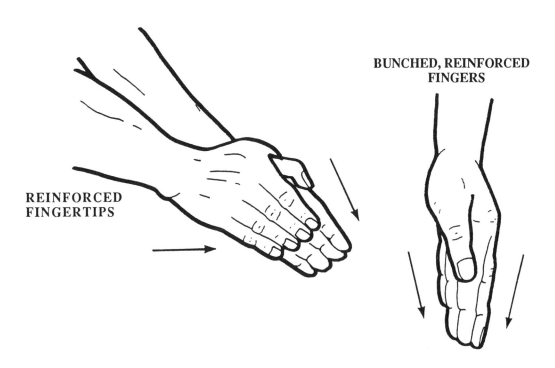

BUNCHED, REINFORCED FINGERS

REINFORCED FINGERTIPS

These strokes are for deep, specific penetration, e.g., quadratus lumborum, iliacus, and pectoralis minor. Keep you fingers arched.

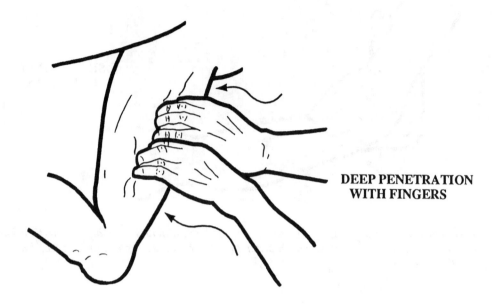

**DEEP PENETRATION
WITH FINGERS**

This illustrates how many deep strokes separate (instead of spreading) tissues which have become stuck together at a deep level. A slow wavelike movement can help this separating.

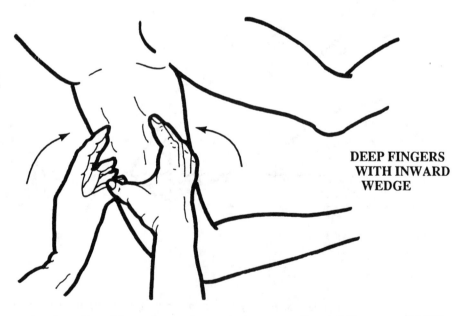

**DEEP FINGERS
WITH INWARD
WEDGE**

Here separation is achieved by a deep, pincer motion, sometimes with an upward lifting movement added.

Chapter VII

FINE ENERGY AND THE FIVE ELEMENTS

In the "Outline of a Session" we saw that working with fine energy is important for preparing, sustaining, and finishing deep tissue work. Let's look now at some specific ways you can regulate fine energy.

GIVING SPACE AND TIME TO YOUR CLIENT

Even if you have no knowledge of acupressure, polarity, or the soft aspects of Reichian work, you can work with fine energy simply by respecting your clients' need to assimilate the changes which you have initiated with deep breathing and deep strokes. Just be there, making yourself available but not intruding on your clients' need to reorient themselves. If they are stuck and need your intervention, you will soon know. Sometimes this waiting should be done without any contact. Sometimes you can gently touch. Place one hand softly on the forehead, the other on the chest (over the heart, e.g.) or on the belly and continue to wait. This will usually have a calming, nurturing effect. Or you may simply hold your client's hand or head.

It is important to give this space and time frequently. Be sure any active expression of anger, fear, etc., however, is finished for the moment, before you begin trying to calm anyone. Cultivate a rhythm in your work in which you feel the need to alternate coarse and fine work. Be ready to stimulate and provoke, or to calm and reassure without pushing your own needs onto the client. This is like riding the waves of change, flowing with ever-changing energy flows.

SIMPLE VERBAL SUPPORT AND DIRECTION

Often simple asking, "How do you feel now," or saying "I know how you feel," or "I have often felt that way too," or "It was good that you let yourself go like that" can give a great deal of support without pushing the person further. (If you are encouraging more active or even explosive expression and release, other types of directives would, of course, be needed).

Fine energy often has to do with seeing, understanding, meditating, watching. After a cathartic release you may want to point out that there are various choices, various routes for letting experience flow. You might, for example, say "It was great to see you express your hate toward your father, and I feel you don't allow that feeling to come out often enough; when you hate him you aren't denying your love; that can be expressed again at another moment." Or "Did you notice how alive you were as you reached out to your mother?" With such questions we are not trying to further confront frustrations, or incomplete feelings, but are merely taking stock of what's happened to this point. Help your clients assimilate their experiences frequently during a session. Avoid discussions about what has happened in the past or theorizing about the human condition. These verbal sidetracks will stop the momentum of the session, and make re- entry into the tissue more difficult.

Another way to direct fine energy is to help your clients formulate a supportive and attainable affirmation. As we saw in Chapter II affirmations, when they remain open ended and are not attempts to manipulate ourselves, are ways for us to claim the power which has been released by the crumbling of our armor. Whenever I repeat to myself, "I am opening myself to the love of other people," my affirmation is broad enough to give me a direction for change. But when I say "I can get Mary to love me," I am manipulating and armoring myself.

If you are working with Gestalt methods, you may find moments when the top dog and underdog have fought to more or less a standstill and are on the verge of sharing, rather than just resistant role playing. At these moments you might encourage your clients to just watch the top dog and underdog. You might also help each side ask the other what it really needs from the other. I have discussed more about the use of Gestalt in Chapter III.

SOME SYSTEMS OF FINE ENERGY

Below is a brief outline of some ways you can use the five elements and acupressure points to regulate fine energy. There are, of course, many other systems which you could effectively use but which we will not discuss. For example, in the Polarity approach there is a careful regulation of the energy of the chakras. Many very powerful points are used simultaneously to connect positive and negative energy. Reflexology, which is a system passing not only through the feet but through the hands and other parts of the body, also provides many useful points for regulating fine energy. Some systems of movement awareness which we have already mentioned in the "Outlining of a Session" are: the Alexander Technique, Feldenkrais Method, and Aston Patterning. Some other equally important ones are Tragering and Pulsing. Although to some extent passive, these help bring the client in touch with a subtle, deep, inner movement.

You will discover the techniques which are best for you as a practitioner. I have chosen to focus on the five elements and acupressure because they come from one of the most rich and flexible systems I know which takes body and mind as a working unity.

THE FIVE ELEMENTS

If you understand the basic flow of energy between the five elements -- water, wood, fire, earth, metal -- you have an orientation which can help you diagnosis and redirect the energy of your clients as you work with breath, emotion and fascia.

Study accompanying five element charts so that you have a sense of the properties and interrelationships between the elements. Also consult Dianne M. Connelly's, Traditional Acupuncture: The Law of the Five Elements, The Centre for Traditional Acupuncture, Inc. The American City Building, Columbia, Maryland 21044.

As you do deep work you will be helping your clients confront the excesses and deficiencies of energy in their five elements. When encountering an excess, e.g., you may wish to provoke the expression of a held back attitude before trying to reorganize tissue. If, for example, someone has an excess of wood energy, I might prod them (with Reichian probes, pokes and scratches) into kicking or slamming out their rage, before trying to move, slowly and deeply, their hardened layers of fascia. As the excess releases in wood, more energy is available in fire to sustain and support lasting bodymind changes. On the other hand, if someone has, for example, a deficiency of metal, I might find it helpful to begin deep tissue work and wait for other elements (fire or earth?) to nurture the hidden sadness. In the first example we have someone who is hard and held back and needs to express themselves before opening up to deep tissue work, whereas in the second example we see tissue which can be entered but needs to be nurtured.

As you work with the five elements you will begin to discover many ways of connecting your knowledge of the five elements with your deep work.

ACUPRESSURE POINTS FOR SESSIONS

1. All Purpose Points. There are number of powerful self- regulating points that you can use at anytime. Self-regulating means that the point will either supply or diminish energy to the elements automatically as needed.

> S36   (Stomach) Leg Three Miles. One of the most powerful all-purpose points in the entire meridian system. Notice that this point is an earth point on an

FIVE ELEMENT ASSOCIATIONS:

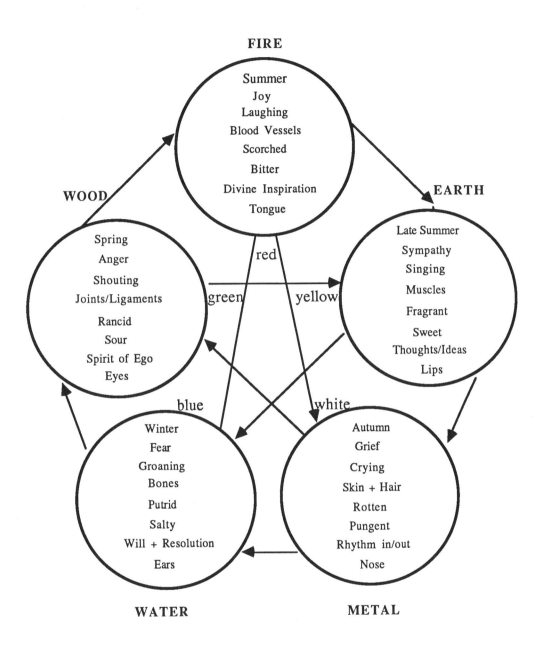

FIRE

Summer
Joy
Laughing
Blood Vessels
Scorched
Bitter
Divine Inspiration
Tongue

WOOD

Spring
Anger
Shouting
Joints/Ligaments
Rancid
Sour
Spirit of Ego
Eyes

EARTH

Late Summer
Sympathy
Singing
Muscles
Fragrant
Sweet
Thoughts/Ideas
Lips

red

green   yellow

blue   white

Winter
Fear
Groaning
Bones
Putrid
Salty
Will + Resolution
Ears

Autumn
Grief
Crying
Skin + Hair
Rotten
Pungent
Rhythm in/out
Nose

WATER   **METAL**

THE 5 ELEMENT CORRESPONDENCES

Element: The 5 moving forces	WOOD	FIRE	EARTH	METAL	WATER
Yin/Yang	young yang	old yang	neutral	young yin	old yin
Direction	east	south	centre	west	north
Season	spring	summer	late summer	autumn	winter
Climate	wind	heat	humidity	dryness	cold
Time of day	morning	midday	afternoon	evening	night
Yin Organs	liver	heart	spleen	lungs	kidneys
Yang Organs	gall bladder	small intest	stomach	colon	bladder
Colours	green	scarlet red	yellow	white	black/blue
Movement	outward	vertical up	horizontal	inward	vertical down
Basic Energetic character	mildly rising warmth	damp-heat	neutralizing and calming	cooling	bitter cold
Astrological animal-YANG	tiger	horse	dog/sheep	rooster	boar
Astrological animal-YIN	hare	serpent	ox/dragon	monkey	rat
A time of	birth	growth	change puberty	maturity/ decline	retention stagnation
Power for	shooting	blossoming	ripening	harvesting	storing
Controls and nourishes the	muscles ligaments	arteries and veins	fleshy musc-les & tone	skin	bones and marrow
Expands into	nails	complexion	lips	body hair	head hair
Sense organ Liquid emitted	eyes tears	tongue sweat	mouth saliva	nose nasal mucous	ears urine
Sense	sight	speech	taste/touch	smell	hearing
Sound	Shouting	laughing	singing	weeping	groaning
Emotion	anger	joy/pleasure	sympathy	sorrow/grief	deep fear
Temperament	depression	up & down	obsession	anguish	fear
Energy type	storage & organization birth	directing influence growth	constructive transforma-tion	rhythmic order harvest	organizational potential hibernation
psychic state	plans, decisions reflections	refinement specif.energy manifestation	collection calming neutralizing	systemic order harmony,rhythm	storage retreat suspension of
Action	wrenching & pulling	blazing flaming act.	cogitation pondering	reservation	trembling or quivering
Element Spirit	soul spiritual faculties ambition	divine spirit love integrity	intellect intelligence ideas memory	animal spirit instinct	will power libido sex drive
Energy type	spiritual	psychic	physical	vital	ancestral
Regulation	development of physic.force	meridians	development of body type	existence of being	imagination & ideas
Specific function potentialization	Planning & reflecting	Cohesion of personality	critical faculty	rhythmic order	of energy
Complexion in illness	olive light green	red & white mixed	yellowish	pale	dark grey-brown

48

	WOOD	FIRE	EARTH	METAL	WATER
Odor emitted in illness	rancid greasy,sour	scorched burnt	fragrant sickly sweet	rotten fishy smoked	putrid decay
When excited patient shows tension release	control holds in	sadness & grief	belching obstinacy	coughs rejected	trembles
In illness beware of	winds	hot food & clothings	big meals damp ground	cold food drink & cloth	scalding food heated clothing
General toxicity	head,weak knees, liver pain,bloodshot eyes	swelling of nose,hands, emotions up & down	drooling, vomiting, ulcers,fat, low energy, obsession	chest congestion, hemorrhoids, anguish, sinus,bowel	hair loss, dandruff, weak ankles, sex probl., painful joints
arthritis,					
Excess	cataracts dizziness insomnia	lazing or flaming action	sweet & greasy taste in perspiration	rapid & deep breath,cracked lips,cough	dry mouth dymphonia excess mucus
Deficiency	headaches depression apprehension nausea	sorrowful demeanor shortness of breath	indigestion diarrhea emaciation heaviness	cold hands & feet cramps	soft speech impotence chills incontinence
Time Excess	worsen 11pm-3am relief 11am-3pm	worsen 11am-3pm relief 11pm-3am	worsen 7am-11am relief 7pm-11pm	worsen 3am-7am relief 3pm-7pm	worsen 3pm-7pm relief 3am-7am
Time Deficiency	worsen 11am-3pm relief 11pm-3am	worsen 11pm-3am relief 11am-3pm	worsen 7pm-11pm relief 7am-11am	worsen 3pm-7pm relief 3am-7am	worsen 3am-7am relief 3pm-7pm
Dream Diagnosis	trees & forests	laughter or fear	chants music, hills,storms,air heaviness	fright,fly, soar through	split between back & waist
Deficiency	lying under tree mushrooms	fire,yang things,hills blazing	lack of food & drink	white objects killing,wars battles	ships boats,drowning
Reversal	fights battles gall bladder	populated towns sm.intestine	eating & drinking stomach	fields rural lg. intest.	walks & travel
bladder					
Flavor	sour	bitter	sweet	pungent	salty
Effect	gathering	strengthening	retarding	dispersing	softening
Opposite	pungent (hot)	salt	sour	bitter	sweet
Effect of Excess	toughens flesh skin	withers ache	bones muscles	knots arteries	hardens
Cereal	wheat,rye	corn	millet	rice,oats	beans,peas
Fruit	plum,berries	apricot	date	peach	grapes
Cooking method	steam	raw	stew	bake	fry
Vegetables	root veg. artichoke beets,celery leek,cabbage	garlic pumpkin chick pea	squash parsnip	comfrey garlic hot pepper	seaweed parsley cabbage
Vitamin	A B-com,K, Folic Acid	Lecithin,C,E, B1,B2,B15	B1,B2 C,E	A,Biotin,D Lecithin	A,C,F,E,D,
To diminish Excess	sage	caraway	basil	garlic,ginger	parsley
To fortify root	licorice	ginseng	orange peel,	cayenne	marshmallow

49

earth meridian which means it reinforces and stabilizes earth, the nurturing element.

Cv17   (Conception Vessel) Within the Breast. This is often called the chi or breath point. Helps in opening breathing, as well as balancing overall energy.

Li4   (Large Intestine) Joining of the Valleys. Although this point is specifically for the colon, throat, and nose, it is also an overall energy regulator and can be especially effective when used with S36.

Sp6   (Spleen) Three Yin Crossing. This point is called the woman's point and affects the ovaries. It should be used frequently since menstruation is often thrown out of it normal cycle. In men this point also has a strong effect on the prostate. Since it is a crossing point of the lower yin meridians its affects the whole length of the inside of the body.

K27   (Kidney) Store House. This is the point for balancing the right and left halves of the body, for harmonizing the masculine and feminine parts of ourselves.

Sp21   (Spleen) Great Enveloping. This point helps balance the energy of the whole thoracic cage.

2. Tonifying Points. If the client needs more energy in a given element and the previous element has an adequate supply, you can use a tonifying point to pull the energy into this deficient element (meridian). For example, if the Gall Bladder is weak and the Bladder is strong -- anger undersupplied, fear excessive -- then use the water point on the Gall Bladder Meridian. Using the point that relates back to the previous element (water, earth, metal points, etc.) you can find the tonifying points for all 12 meridians. I list only some of these tonification points below as well as some other stimulating points.

H9   (Heart) Little Rushing In. Since the fire element has four meridians -- heart, small intestine, circulation, and triple warmer -- supplying energy to this element has a strong overall tonifying effect to the whole system. Fire is the great coordinator and regulator of the whole meridian system so be careful not to overstimulate.

Li11   (Large Intestine) Crooked Pond. This tonifying point is especially effective when used with S36.

Gv14   (Governing Vessel) The Great Hammer. This point is a judo revival point and can be hit with a glancing, crisp blow to bring back the energy of a client who is falling into a lethargic, unresponsive state.

Lv8   (Liver) Crooked Spring. This point is good for stimulating the capacity to build and maintain assertiveness -- not explosive anger, but steady initiative.

B67   (Bladder) Extremity of Yin. The bladder meridian is the longest meridian. Stimulating this point will bring energy down the whole length of the back of the body.

H3   (Heart) Little Sea or the Joy of Life. This point stimulates fire but at the same time calms water. It turns fear into joy.

3. Sedating Points. If the client has an excess of energy in an element (meridian), you can disperse this excess by using a sedating point to send this excess on to the next element (meridian), assuming the next meridian is not already overloaded. For example, if my client has excessive fire in the heart meridian (too joyful, nervously overactive), and needs more nurturing earth energy, I can use the earth point on the heart meridian to reduce fire and supply earth, diminish joy and increase sympathy. All twelve sedation points can be found by taking the point which relates to the next meridian in the five element cycle. I list some of these, as well as other calming points.

> K1   (Kidney) Bubbling Spring. This point not only calms but has a harmonizing effect upon the sympathetic and parasympathetic nervous systems. After the intense upheaval and release during a session, these systems can be out of balance. We may be sympathetically overstimulated, or parasympathetically lethargic (as a defensive reaction).

> H7   (Heart) Spirit Gate. Very strong sedating point. Note that earth, which by nature is nurturing, will be further nurtured. Neighboring points, H4, 5, and 6 can help with speech which is too rapid or tongue tied. To calm oneself is to find the door to one's spirit and capacity to speak with one's heart.

> CS7   (Circulation Sex) The Great Mound. This point has been used for extreme nervousness.

> Gb34 (Gall Bladder) Yang Mound Spring. This point is good against muscular cramping. Helps relax the entire musculature. You can use it just before deep, difficult strokes.

4. Points for Pelvic Release. Doors of Life. These points are in an area which is very active during birth. Often in a rebirthing session massage of this area prompts a reliving of birth itself.

> Gv4   (Governing Vessel) Gate of Life. Locate by drawing a line horizontal between the twelfth ribs and crests of each ilium.

> B23   (Bladder) Kidneys Correspondence.

> B47   (Bladder) Ambition Room.

> Groin and Genitals

> S30   (Stomach) Rushing Order. Located right along the superior line of the pubic bone. Erotically stimulating.

> Lv10   (Liver) Five Miles.

> Lv11   (Liver) Yin Angle.

> Lv12   (Liver) Hasty Pulse.

5. Windows to the Sky. These points bring energy upward. When working on the upper half of the body, they can supply energy taken from the lower half. After having worked on the lower half of the body, you can also balance out the effect by returning energy to the upper half with these points.

Cs1   (Circulation Sex) Heavenly Pond.

Cv22 (Conception Vessel) Heaven Rushing Out.

Li18 (Large Intestine) Support and Rush Out.

S9   (Stomach) People Welcome.

Si16 (Small Intestine) Heavenly Window.

Si17 (Small Intestine) Heavenly Appearance.

Tw16 (Triple Warmer) Heavenly Window.

B10   (Bladder) Heavenly Pillar.

Gv16 (Governing Vessel) Wind Palace.

L3   (Lung) Heavenly Palace.

6. Points in Areas Covered by Sessions. During the session you will be working in areas of the body where there are points which can help you open and relax the structure before making your strokes.

L1   (Lung) Middle Palace.

L2   (Lung) Cloud Gate. These first two lung points open the upper chest.

Lv14 (Liver) Gate of Hope. This point helps elongate the belly.

Gb25 (Gall Bladder) Capital Gate. Opens the back of waist. It is also an alarm point for the kidneys.

Gb29 (Gall Bladder) Dwelling in the Bone.

Gb30 (Gall Bladder) Jumping Circle. These two Gall Bladder points release the lateral hip and iliotibial tract.

K10   (Kidney) Yin Valley. Water point on a water meridian. Stores and stabilizes energy.

B50   (Bladder) Receive and Support. This point connects the legs and pelvis.

B54   (Bladder) Equilibrium Middle. Earth point on water. Brings sympathy into fear. Helps knees be more flexible and supportive.

Gb20 (Gall Bladder) Wind Pond. Releases excess aggressive energy which collects at the base of occiput.

Chapter VIII

BODYMIND TYPES AND THE LIMITS OF CHANGE

Guiding Without Classifying

When healing change is seen as a reciprocal exchange between practitioner and individual, the dilemma we faced at the beginning of this chapter is resolved. When I give my force, feelings, and ideas to you from a receptive and unified inner and outer space, I am simultaneously allowing you to explore your own energy. Whenever I "read" you as belonging to a certain bodymind type or structure, I am respecting your capacity to break the limits of this classification and to find your own limits.

A number of bodyworkers and therapists have explored a wide variety of physical and psychological types. In **Know Your Type** (4) Ralph Metzner outlines and summarizes a selection of types, including those of Sheldon (mesomorph, endomorph, and ectomorph); Kurtz (bottom-heavy, top-heavy, burdened, rigid, and needy types); and Jung (introvert and extrovert). He also gives various psychiatric types from Freud, Reich, and Lowen, and the classic western types (choleric, sanguine, phlegmatic, and melancholic). Rather than a further review of these types, I offer a classification system which has evolved from my work over the years. My schema is intended to supplement and not replace the types specified by Metzner and is designed to be flexible in providing individuals with a framework which allows interaction with the practitioner.

This schema does not try to classify the individual directly but indicates that some detectable characteristics or structure may belong to a type or number of types. This gives a starting point from which the individual can be expressive, without being treated as an object. For example, instead of indicating that you are a "burdened type," I may share with you that your shoulders look heavy, and ask you how you feel in your shoulders. With this kind of shared impression and interrogation our interaction can more likely develop into a discovery of what you feel and want and what I, in turn, can give to you.

Exchange the following with a friend:

> **Face each other and share what you see in each other's structure. Be sure to ask if your partner feels that your impression is true. Encourage an exploration of the feeling and thoughts in various parts of the body by exaggerating the position or exploring an alternative position. Try out a type which you resemble (top-heavy, bottom-heavy, etc.) by saying, for example, both: "I am top heavy," and "I am not only top-heavy," that is, affirm that part of the classification you accept and deny what you don't accept.**

We may discover in the process of interacting and sharing that what is happening in your shoulders is of less importance to your release and integration than what is happening in other parts of your structure. We may discover that a feeling of neediness around your mouth and throat is equally significant as, or even more significant than, my initial observation about your shoulders.

Type consideration is merely a suggested starting point for discovery and transformation. After the client moves through his or her process of transformation, we can then look back and consider the degree of change and how much movement has been made away from the type with which we started. Now that there has been change, the client, for example may no longer be very much like a "needy" type, he or she may be fuller, softer, and more expanded, and more closely resemble what I presently shall describe as an "even" type. This flexible approach to types allows a discovery of limitations and a decision about what one wants to accept or work to overcome.

BODYMIND TYPES

TYPE	OUTSIDE STRUCTURE, SHELL	INSIDE INTRINSIC STRUCTURE	FUNCTION	COMPARISON TO OTHER TYPES
I. EXPANDING outer directed		United Core		
A. SOFT	LOOSE: superficial tissue available, fat porous, voluminous; reaction is slow but responsive	TIGHT: hidden, frozen, immobile	Outer sleeve is protective cushion for unused inner energy	Extrovert who hides inner feeling, bottomheavy, seductive, rigid inside, paralyzed paranoic, masochistic, burdened, endomorph
B. HARD	TIGHT: thick skinned, muscular, dense, quick voluminous, massive	LOOSE: little tone, weak, confused, underdeveloped	Strong, active exterior covers fragile inner energy	Extrovert with little inner development, topheavy, manipulative, sadist, rigid outside, mesomorph
II. CONTRACTING inner directed		DUAL CORE — Outer Core / Inner Core		
A. HARD	TIGHT OR LOOSE: Unconscious, unresponsive, rubbery, fronzen, stoic	TIGHT: Both are underdeveloped	Lack of outside consciousness compensated by active introverted energy	Active introvert, phlegmatic outside, choleric inside, compulsive, anal, ectomorph
B. Soft	LOOSE: unconscious, unresponsive, rubbery, fronzen, stoic	TIGHT: outer core restricts inner core LOOSE: inner core is weak and fragile	Inner activity is not well directed	Confused introvert, needy, oral, masochist, melancholic, burdened, endomorph, hysteric
III. UNSTABLE excess inside or outside				
A. OVEREXTENDING				
1. CONTRACTING	STABLE	TIGHT: Entire Core is Overactive or TIGHT: Outer Core Traps Inner	Under stress energy is focused inside or outside for protection	Part time introvert or part time extrovert, neurotic, body changes frequently
2. EXPANDING	LOOSE: overconscious or unresponsive TIGHT: overprotective	STABLE		
B. FLUCTUATING	UNSTABLE	UNSTABLE	Unpredictable and excessive movement toward both expansion and contraction	Schizoid, manic depressive, hysteric, oscillating mixture of many types
IV. EVEN equal tone				
A. HARD EVEN	TIGHT	TIGHT	Even but excessive tone; too protective in both shell and core	Has capacity to be open but holds back some of energy
B. SOFT EVEN	LOOSE	LOOSE	Even but inadequate tone; too open in both shell and core	Has capacity to conserve energy, but gives away too much
C. BALANCED	OPEN TO CHANGE	BALANCED: outside and inside is even; shell and core disappear	Allows energy to flow to where it is needed	Genital, spontaneous, loving, both open and self-protective

Jonathan was a professor of philosophy. His body was lean, small-boned and somewhat boyish and fragile, while his head was relatively large and pointed. He had been trying to gain weight for years by lifting weights and taking protein supplements, and although his muscles had tightened, he had not become much larger.

As I started working with him, I expected a softening and balancing of his body but no major changes in his size. I encouraged him to stop heavy exercise, pointing out that his body was close to what Sheldon has classified as ectomorph (thin body, large head, lack of muscular development). After I had worked with him for seven sessions, I was surprised that he looked much larger, much more expanded in his musculature; even his bones seemed to have grown.

He shared with me that during the previous week he had a flashback memory, which he felt through his whole self. He remembered that at the age of five he was unable to compete with his brothers in feats of physical strength and skill and so he had turned to mental activity in an attempt to gain the approval of his parents. Yet he still felt insecure and had started lifting weights in an attempt to prove to himself he was really powerful. After seven sessions, he realized he did not have to compete but could explore his physical strength in other ways. He began enjoying swimming, running, and dancing.

During the next six months, as I completed the remaining three sessions, he expanded two inches around his chest, and his thigh and calf muscles became full but soft. And even his head was less pointed. I was happily surprised that he went far beyond the limits I had initially envisaged for him.

Early in life we begin to develop our strength and consciousness by concentrating more on the outside or more on the inside of ourselves. In so doing we armor ourselves in characteristic ways that resemble what I call "expanding" and "contracting" types of bodymind. When we fluctuate unevenly between outside and inside, we may resemble what I call an "unstable" type. When our inner and outer rhythms are somewhat equal, we may resemble what I want to call an "even" type. Even when the range of expansion and contraction is to a certain extent restricted, we may still be close to an even type.

The following classifications evolved more from tactile than visual cues, so are difficult to illustrate, except in the accompanying crosssections of the body. They also cut across previous classifications, that is to say, one of my types may be similar to more than one traditional type. The chart provided is not complete or definitive, but I hope it suggests to you examples of such types from your own experience.

EXPANDING TYPES

Taking Up Outer Space

We have moods in which we are outgoing, in which we make contact with the people around us or the objects in our environment. In this external movement we may be enthusiastic and filled with vitality and purpose, or quiet, slow, and not so clearly directed. There are many individuals who focus the main part of their lives on this extroverted dimension and who in some ways neglect the inner side of themselves. They display a kind of expanding, well-developed outer armor or defense in dealing with life. The chart shows two possible expanding types: a soft one, which is loose outside and tight inside, and a hard one, which is tight outside and loose inside.

The first kind of expanding person has developed a loose outer sleeve around the body (mind), providing a soft, fat, porous protection for absorbing the pains, demands, shocks, and tensions of everyday life. Although this large, elastic surface creates a broad, flexible contact with the world and other people, it is a shell, a kind of cushion, allowing the individual to react from the outside, perhaps slowly, without expressing the more contracted inner feelings. The inside remains frozen and mostly unconscious, used only when the individual is touched deeply, or when called upon to use his or her reserve strength.

Whenever I am working with a person whose tissue and personality show some of these traits, I explore the direction of our work together by either provoking the person outside, encouraging a quicker response to me, or by trying to work my way slowly through the soft, outer shell to the evasive deepest tissue, feelings, and thoughts.

> **Maria, from Florence, had been married to her domineering husband ten years. She was obedient to him, but was not at all timid, and managed to go around him when she really wanted something to which he was opposed. She was not very fat but rather large in the hips and upper thighs. Her tissue was spongy and rubbery and she had little feeling on the surface and at the intermediate level of tissue. As I worked I had to hook the tissue sharply with my fingers, take up any slack, and hold my grip encouraging her to breathe more rapidly and to make loud sounds as she exhaled. Gradually, with each session, she began to respond faster, and to understand that it was o.k. for her to let her deeper feelings come to the surface.**

The second kind of expanding type is muscular, massive, dense, or thick-skinned. These individuals also use their body volume as a protection device. Since they are tight outside, they can take, and even enjoy, more rough contact to the point of aggressive interaction with others. Although their reactions may be quicker, they remain superficial unless the hard shell is broken or dissolved. I try forceful, aggressive encounter with such hard shelled individuals, or else I try circumventing their outer armor with gentleness, encouraging them to expose their looser, inner selves. In either strategy, when the outside armor begins to disappear, I find it helpful to explore ways of keeping the often confused, underdeveloped interior intact with guided movements, and slow, careful initiation into new attitudes.

> **Tony was an English "skin head." He considered himself tough and ready to confront the authorities or rowdies who were not part of his gang. Underneath he was actually very needy. In the first sessions he wanted to express his anger as fully as possible. I supported this by provoking him with words and quick taps on the belly, but I waited for the moment he would accept more gentle work. During the fourth session after he had exploded with anger and was trembling in exhaustion, I rocked him softly and sang a lullaby. As he began sobbing I was able, without much pressure, to begin moving through previously resistant layers of tissue.**

You can look at yourself in relation to the expanding types with the following:

> **Do you consider yourself to be ample and soft on the outside of your body? Can you easily grasp the flesh of your thighs between your thumb and forefinger? When you squeeze hard to you feel any pain? Consider whether you**

have a rather soft and unconscious protective buffer on the outside of your body. If you see yourself as soft and expanding, do you also see that at a deeper level you have a lot of resistance?

Do you think of yourself as rather large and tight on the surface? Is it difficult to pinch the flesh on your thighs? Do you like a lot of vigorous activities like running, swimming, dancing? Did you fight or wrestle with other children when you were a child? If you consider yourself as hard and expanding, reflect on whether you are clear about your inner feelings, and whether you find, it easy to be alone, to meditate quietly.

CONTRACTING TYPES

Busy Inner Worlds

Whereas the life of the expanding type is filled with outer contact, the contracting individual withdraws and holds back from external engagement and interaction. These individuals perhaps appear calm on the surface, but underneath create conscious, active, and tense inner movements (which contrasts with the frozen inactivity of the soft, expanding type who is also tight inside).

This inner activity takes two forms. First in the hard, contracting type, the entire core structure is overactive and the shell neglected, as in the case of the person who is continually avoiding any outer contact by a frenzy of inner movement. Here the outside may be relatively loose but lacking in the receptivity of the slow, conscious responsiveness of the soft expanding type.

Second, the soft contracting type has a contraction of the deep extrinsic muscles (which we can classify as the periphery of the core), surrounding the even deeper intrinsic muscles (the inner core). The contraction of the relatively deep extrinsic muscles (peripheral core) traps the deeper intrinsic muscles (inner core) and restricts their mobility and power. (We saw in previous chapters how the psoas can be overpowered by surrounding structures). The outer core is, then, tight and overdeveloped, while the inner core is loose, inactive, and weak. This soft contracting type differs from the hard expanding type (who is also loose inside) in that in this type the shell is loose and relatively lacking in energetic response.

With both contracting types I encourage exploration and use of their external power -- the expression of anger, joy, enthusiasm, the open display of thoughts and feelings. With the second type, however, since the inner and outer extremes are weak (the shell and inner core are soft), I suggest that their outer movements and expressions be slow and careful explorations,accompanied by subtle, conscious inner attitudes.

First an example of a hard contracting type:

Sagarito was a religious devotee who meditated twice a day. He was always disciplining his thoughts and feelings, seeking purity and enlightenment. He felt that his body was only a vehicle to be used to help advance his spiritual aspirations. The outside of his body, although not hard like a hard expanding type, was rather lifeless. He was quiet and responsive as I pressed through the outer layers, then as I reached deeper he would stop me, saying he found that there were overwhelming images and sensations which he could not assimilate. I found the most effective way to work with him was to keep my hands at an intermediate depth, and invite him to decide when I was to go deeper. As I waited for his acceptance, I encouraged him not only to verbally express his images and feelings, but also to translate these into movements in his legs, arms, and head.

Here's an example of a soft contracting type:

> Sorgen was a Danish economic professor in Copenhagen. He was rather soft on the surface and was very sincere and interested in others. But he had a theory about everybody he met and was continually intervening in other people's disputes, interpreting their attitudes toward each other. He stayed busy with these ideas, but when pressed, found it difficult to express any feelings of his own -- he would become confused if not allowed to talk about others.
>
> In the later sessions of work, as I began waking up his deep intrinsic muscles, I encouraged him not to think or verbally express himself, but to pantomime in slow motion his attitude toward his father, mother, and toward himself. These slow movements with exaggerated facial expressions helped him begin to focus on very concrete, simple feelings inside himself.

Find your relation to contracting types with the following:

> Do you feel tight in the center of your body? Do you spend a lot of your time making decisions, fantasizing, or just thinking things over? Are you so busy that you sometimes do not notice that you have bruised or cut yourself? As a test of whether you are a hard contracting type consider whether you can totally relax, both outside and inside.
>
> Do you keep your mind occupied, so that you won't have time to get upset? Do you use a soft, pleasant even accommodating attitude toward others to cover up your doubts and inner confusions? Do these uncertainties take a lot of your energy? If you feel that you, at least in part, fit the soft contracting type, notice how difficult it may be to make a simple decision and to carry it out, without delay or problems.

UNSTABLE TYPES

Over The Edge And Swinging Back And Forth

Some individuals easily change the direction of their energy and awareness between inside and outside so that they are not stuck in either, yet make these changes as a result of their instability and not in harmony with their needs and environment. There are two kinds of instability. One results from overextension of the self, and the other from disruptive fluctuation within the self.

Overextension is toward expansion or toward contraction. These individuals may be usually balanced in their outer and inner activity, but under stress, they focus too much of their energy either outward or inward. They may have no problem with one half of their lives. If they sometimes exhaust themselves in expanding, they may not have a corresponding degree in contracting, and though inclined to withdraw into themselves, they may still manage to cope with outside demands. Their weakness is in one direction, and unlike the previous expanding and contracting types, they can eventually, even if temporarily, regain a balance between inside and outside.

> Georgia seemed like a lady who successfully handled her life. She had graduated from college and had a good paying job as a junior executive in a large firm. She was

58

> outgoing, pleasant, and efficient. But after six months of
> marriage her world fell apart. Her life had been built
> around control and discipline, but she was unable to
> control her husband the way she had controlled her life.
> She became very nervous, unsure of herself, and withdrawn.

The second kind of instability is seen in the individual who, perhaps wildly, fluctuates between extremes. These persons are unpredictably expanding in one moment and contracting in the next. Typical would be the person who gains excessive weight in a matter of days or weeks, and loses it just as quickly. This could be the manic-depressive, now joyful and overflowing, and then suddenly gravely depressed. We all expand and contract. However, depending upon the extent we are balanced and flowing, we exercise a centered and spontaneous choice about the timing, degree, and rate of our expansions and contractions.

> Whenever Tim was encouraged to express himself, he
> fell silent and withdrew his energy. Whenever anyone tried
> to calm him, he became more nervous and active. Sometimes
> when I worked with him I could press deep into his tissue
> without him reacting, and then suddenly without warning
> he would contract and jerk away.

Both unstable types show an unevenness in tissue and attitudes. They may collapse under pressure, into a slack, disorganized state. Or if they are touched deeply, they may pull together in an over-contracting defense. In consideration of these fragilities, I have found it important to work with these individuals in a nonprovocative and predictable manner, helping them learn that change can be safe, gradual, and progressive.

Compare yourself to these unstable types with the following:

> Do you find that your body is strong and stable for months
> at a time, and then suddenly you find yourself weak and
> collapsing? Are you a quiet, withdrawn person who surprises
> everybody by becoming the outgoing life of the party? Do you
> consider yourself unstable because you overextend yourself?
>
> Do you sometimes think that you have radically different
> personalities which you can't control? Do you feel that there
> is no real you, but just different roles you play? Do the
> proportions of your body change enough for you to consider
> yourself to be in some respects an unstable fluctuating type?

EVEN TYPES

Staying Consistent And Flexible

There exist those rare individuals who balance their expanding and contracting sides, their outer and inner selves, and who change with their environment, but not because of it. They have bodyminds whose outer, intermediate, and deepest layers are all more or less equal in tonus, flexibility, and responsiveness. Their bodyminds have little in the way of a protective core and shell, since they are able to mobilize their entire selves when threatened from within or without. As previously stated in Chapter II:

> When we are really alive, the core and shell
> disintegrate; our energy moves easily from outside to
> inside and from inside to outside. There is a balance
> between the larger extrinsic muscles which give power to
> our movements and the inner intrinsic muscles, which give
> subtle direction and stability.

When subjected to severe stress for long periods of time, even types may tend to protect themselves, by equally restricting the range of both expansion and contraction, but not by losing their balance between inside and outside. I find them most satisfying to work with, since their transformations are rapid and smooth. Compare this kind of balanced change with the changes of expanding types, who are slow in responding to probes into their soft buffer or who melt in confusion as their hard exterior breaks open; or with the changes of contracting types, who stubbornly resist deep, gentle surrender; and with the uneven types who keep changing directions to avoid confrontation.

> Hassad was a Lebanese businessman who often visited Europe. He was sanguine and friendly and had a well-proportioned body whose tissues were soft, yet responsive from the outside to even the deepest layers. I had, over a period of a year, given him more than ten sessions of work on his visits to Paris. At about this time the Lebanese civil war worsened, and on his next visit I found him tight and afraid for the safety of his family.
> At this point it took only one session to soften and balance his body. He cried a lot and expressed his anger against the war. He himself wanted to leave Lebanon but his large family wanted to stay, and he had made the decision to stay with them.
> When I met him again six months later in Paris, he was again contracted and afraid. But again he was able to let go quickly and express his feelings.

You can get a feeling for the even type by considering the following:

> Reflect on a time in your life when you were happy for an extended period of time. Remember how you were able to ride out your difficulties without losing your sense of well being. Remember how you were able to express different feelings freely, even anger and sadness, without getting stuck in them. Remember the health and resilience of your body, how sickness was a temporary cleansing of the body. Compare this happy period with a period in which you were blocked and unhappy.

In working with each individual, I recognize that a type is a stereotype, and that we are only looking for starting and comparison points. Each person will respond differently to the above suggested ways of exploring and working with different types. The same individual may even react differently at different times. That is why I keep making new suggestions, posing new questions, trying to discover new ways of making contact with each individual and in the process find that I am changing myself.

PART II

TECHNICAL SUMMARY OF TEN SESSIONS

OF DEEP BODYWORK

THE PROCESS OF RELEASE AND INTEGRATION

	SEGMENTS AND MUSCULATURE	FASCIAE	ATTITUDES, MOVEMENTS, FEELINGS
FIRST STAGE: Release of Armor in Individual Bodymind Segments			
PHASE I: Initial Opening of Bodymind Armor	Balancing the outside: upper and lower structures	Superficial envelop	Surface feelings, momentary reactions, habitual defenses
SESSION 1: Upper Half	Thorax, arms, lateral hips, iliotibial tract, ischia, neck, dorsal and lumbar spine	Superficial pectoralis, abdominus, capitae, colli, nuchae, axillaris, extremitatis superioris	Feelings of being energized or relieved
SESSION 2: Lower Half	Feet, ankles, lower legs, knees, hamstrings, connections to upper half	Superficial extremitatis inferior	Memories of childhood mobility and freedom, grounding, attitudes toward parents
PHASE II: Elongation	Distance between pelvis and cage, shaping (ovality) of thorax, placement of shoulders	Intermediate fascia, superficial part of deep envelopes	Vulnerability along the flanks
SESSION 3: Hips to Shoulders	Hips, cage, shoulders & neck, quad lumborum, lat dorsi, rotators of arms, trapezius	Profunda: dorsi, lumbodorsalis, axillaris, scapulae, nuchae	Increased consciousness in back, lateral mobility enhanced
PHASE III: Pelvic Reorientation	Bottom and front of lower pelvis, top of pelvis and abdomen, back of pelvis and lower back	Deep envelopes around and inside of pelvis	Discovery of central balance, hara consciousness
SESSION 4: Lower Pelvis	Inside of thighs, adductors, front of thighs, rectus femoris, sartorius	Deepest envelopes of adductors, full release of fascia lata	Opening and widening of ischia, lengthening in front, confrontation with sexual feelings
SESSION 5: Upper Pelvis	Abdominus rectus, chest, diaphragm, obliques, psoas	Profunda: scarpa, transversalis, pelvia; envelopes and attachments of ilio-psoas	Settling of abdominal contents into pelvic bowl; joy, sadness, sexual mobility
SESSION 6: Back of Pelvis	Hamstrings, gluteals, rotators, sacrum, sacrospinalis, coccyx	Profunda: lata, pelvia dorsi, envelopes of piriformis, gemelli; obturators, quadratus femoris	Anal anger, male fear of homosexuality, extroverted energy
PHASE IV: Release of Neck And Head			
SESSION 7: Neck and Head	Clavicle, thoracic inlet, neck, scalp, jaw, mouth, tongue, cheeks, nose, eyes	Profunda: nuchae, colli, capitis	Primitive emotions of face, deep pain and release; increase in range of rotation of head
SECOND STAGE: Integration Of All Parts And Aspects Of Bodymind	Connecting segments	All layers move simultaneously	New balance, feeling of wholeness, flowing of emotions and thoughts
PHASE V: Coordinating Upper And Lower Halves	Coordination of either lower or upper segments with each other	Planes of fasciae on opposite half are opened	Feeling of deep opening toward the top or bottom
SESSION 8: Usually Lower Half	Freeing of pelvis and lower extremities	Lifting and lengthening fascia of trunk out of pelvic bowl as result of work on lower half	Feeling that grounding and consciousness in lower half are necessary to freedom above
SESSION 9: Usually Upper Half	Expansion of trunk and upper extremities	Expansion of diaphragmatic fascia downward and outward	Feeling that expression of freedom and needs in upper body helps grounding
SESSION 10: Overall Reorganization	Coordination and connection from front to back and left to right	Freedom and interplay of all fascial layers	Feeling of completeness; front-back, and left-right balance

PHASE I: INITIAL OPENING OF BODYMIND

Sessions 1 and 2

GENERAL PURPOSE

At the outset we want to help our clients feel that they can and will change. This is a inspirational session which communicates the feeling of a fresh and powerful beginning with the promise of more changes to come. We will be releasing superficial fascia, and surface emotions and attitudes. The focus will be on more freedom for the rib cage, shoulders, neck and hips to move in their large superficial fascial envelops. At the same time it is important to do sufficient deep work (e.g., gag and cough reflexes, massage of abdominal contents) for the deep, inner energy to surface and make this superficial work easier. Be careful to not do more deep work than your client can assimilate in initial bodywork.

We want to encourage the large superficial myofascial envelope to expand, to separate from deeper layers, to fluff out, to give room for underlying structures, or where this envelope is too
loose, to encourage more response and contraction. We also want to build the energy level to a point where basic problems can be confronted. In cases where energy is excessive to encourage discharge of pent up feelings and begin to work with underlying needs.

BODYTYPE

1. Hard Outside, Soft Inside. When the outside is hard, the practitioner can either a) work with force to break directly through the superficial armor (in which case enough attention has also to be given to the underlying deeper structures which are soft, disorganized and confused) or b) work subtly to activate deeper feelings which can in turn allow the superficial surface to soften and become more receptive.

2. Soft Outside, Hard Inside. When the outside is soft or rubbery more twisting and hooking of the superficial tissue may be needed. Rubbery types can usually withstand a great deal of superficial manipulation without feeling much discomfort. Slapping, pinching, scratching, tickling may be called for when the exterior is unresponsive. More response in the tissue and feelings is needed, before the slower systematic work can be effective. Soft types who bruise easily may be using their fragility as a protection against deep work. Go slowly, reassure them, but work deep enough.

3. Top Heavy. When this type lacks consciousness in the pelvis and legs, one may begin on the lower half first, or if you find it important to begin working with the rib cage in order to encourage better breathing, then combine, in the same session, at least some work on the legs.

4. Burdened and Needy. These types may require extra work on the belly and chest, while many Rigid types may need more work on the back of the neck and in the middle of the back.

5. Compulsive-Obsessive. Be sure in initial sessions not to pressure these types. They need to be confronted eventually, to have their game exposed, but can easily be frightened away in the beginning. (They will not, of course, admit their fear).

EMOTION

It is not essential that very deep feelings be released during this session (if they arise, certainly give space for them to complete themselves); often playful or extroverted feel-

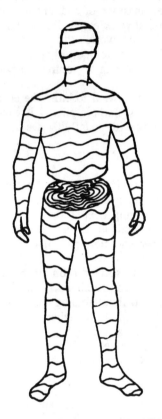 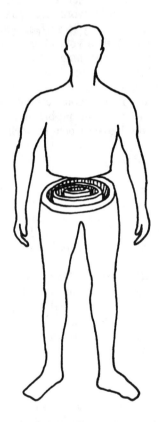

The body can be viewed as similar to an onion with layers of tissue. But this view tends to reinforce the idea that we are made up of parts which need to be released separately and individually. Actually, the body is more like a vibrant, plastic mass, less viscous in some places than others, but made up of the same interflowing stuff. When touched at any level or depth, it instantaneously responds, reshaping itself in every other dimension and part.

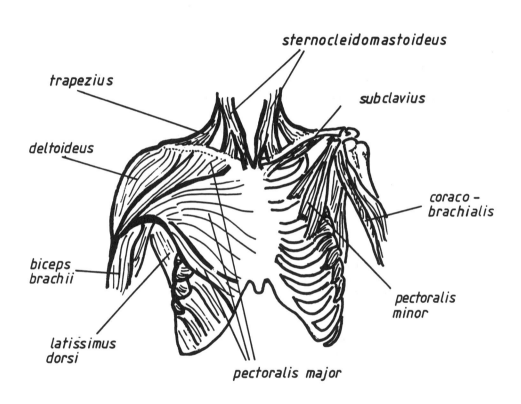

sternocleidomastoideus

trapezius

subclavius

deltoideus

coraco-
brachialis

biceps
brachii

pectoralis
minor

latissimus
dorsi

pectoralis major

ings, attitudes, and movements will be enough of a preparation for deeper feelings to be expressed in later sessions. Confrontation may be more appropriate in later sessions; whereas light and positive affirmations may be easier for the client to assimilate at this point. Remember what is superficial to the practitioner may be deep enough for the client.

If the client, however, is not responsive enough for there to be movement of superficial structures, some deep work around the jaw, in the nose, or with the gag or cough reflexes may help get an overall reaction started, then the superficial tissue will be more receptive. We are not peeling an onion (that is, working only on the outside) but helping the individual make connections between the surface and interior feelings.

THOUGHT AND AFFIRMATION

Many clients may realize, for the first time, that their old thought patterns were limited to considering that either this or that is the only choice. The release of tissue opens new possibilities for them which can be supported and affirmed. For example, "I can begin completely fresh," (that is without the past), "I can handle my pain," (without armor), "I can open myself," "It's o.k. to be afraid (angry sad, happy)."

MANIPULATIONS

1. Broad strokes. Just below the skin help to distribute areas of bunched superficial fascia. Working too deep, too soon, may confuse the complicated myofascial structures.

2. Two handed strokes can help broadly distribute tissue.

3. Hooking, twisting, and spinning may be needed with fingers, elbows, knuckles, or sides of hands in order to capture hard or evasive tissue.

4. Follow the contours of the outer surface of the body. Do not try to imagine the underlying myofascial structures which envelope individual muscles.

5. Focus on seams, where connective tissue attaches to bones or is thickened around tendons and ligaments, such as the mid-line of the breast bone, the edge of ribs along the line of the diaphragmatic arch, either side of the vertebral column, the iliotibial tract, the inner and outer edges of the tibia, the contours of the inner and outer malleolus. Do not try to penetrate to these attachments, but deal with the thick areas of superficial tissue over them.

6. Strokes are generally transverse, across the underlying muscular structures. Work across the grain lengthens the structure. Think of plucking across a guitar string. This is especially true of later, deeper work.

BREATH AND ENERGY WORK

1. The first phase is an exploration of the individual's need for more charge or discharge. Experiment with building energy through inhalation or releasing excessive charge through exhalation. Let this be experimental and playful. Do not begin tissue work until there is some equality in incoming and outgoing energy.

2. During the first phase it may be better to back away from hyperventilation, which can be a frightening experience for many people; later they will be better prepared to go through the accompanying cramps by fully experiencing their fear or hidden anger. If both of you are ready to go through the hyperventilation, then encourage, movement and the expression of feelings locked in the hands and mouth.

3. When working with excessively charged or discharged individuals, it may be important to encourage them to run the course of their excessive breathing pattern, before suggesting that they focus on the neglected aspect of their breathing. For example a highly charged person may need to charge even more, to the point of an explosion, before you can guide him or her to a gentle way of charging, and an undelayed way of discharging.

4. Some exercises that will be good for the first session (See Chapter IV, "Breath and Energy Flow": Those for overall energy flow (The Bow, Between Heaven and Earth, Forward Bend, Wood Chopper); Panting (Chest and Belly).

MOVEMENT AWARENESS

Emphasize extrinsic movements of the arms and legs. During the first sessions it is especially important that the client compares the new freedom of one side of the body with the deadness and stiffness of the untouched side. Although you can start teaching the intrinsic use of the psoas (rolling of the pelvis with inhalation), it is only during later deep work that an actual manipulation of the intrinsic muscles is possible. Interaction with the model is essential in helping create maximum change. The first step will be to get relaxation and surrender from the individual; overeagerness to help or anticipation of what's to come will work against complete change. After you have found the right depth and begin to hook the superficial tissue, ask for an appropriate but gentle movement, or at least a slight contraction of the muscles. Be sure the model is using only the muscles needed for change toward a more balanced structure. We want to help isolate the awareness and function of different muscle groups.

MERIDIANS AND POINTS

Check to see if there is a general concentration of energy in the upper half (overinflated chest, overeager contracted arms; large, stiff neck; red, explosive face) or lower half of the body (contracted medial arches, bow legs with overdeveloped thighs; puffy ankles or knees with water retention). Before and during the session in question, brush the meridians which terminate where there is less energy. For example if the chest is weak and collapsed, brush the lower yin meridians (spleen, kidneys, and liver) upward to the chest and continue this circulation of energy by brushing the upper, inner yin meridians (heart, circulation, lungs). In the upper half of the body general points to be used are: Cv 17, Sp 21, Li 4, Liv 14. In the lower half: S 36, Sp 6, S 41, Liv 10, 11, 12, Gb 25, 29, 30; Water points on inner knee {Liv 8, K10, Sp 9).

CHAKRAS

The focus of the first session is around the heart and throat centers. We want to encourage openness and receptivity. Be sure not to push your client's aggression beyond the capacity of these centers to assimilate and absorb change in a nurturing and self-loving way. The second session on the lower half will activate the basal chakra, and as long as there has already been some opening around the heart will send a charge upward in the body. Use Polarity or acupuncture points to help bring about a balancing of these centers. Using meditation bells and quiet chanting of om can help.

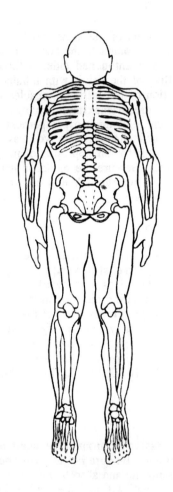

When the rib cage is free, it appears to float like a parachute, and the pelvis and legs lightly dangle below. The bodyweight is then evenly distributed throughout the structure and is supported by the myofascial (tissue) network, rather than bearing down on the spine, pelvis, and bones of the legs and feet.

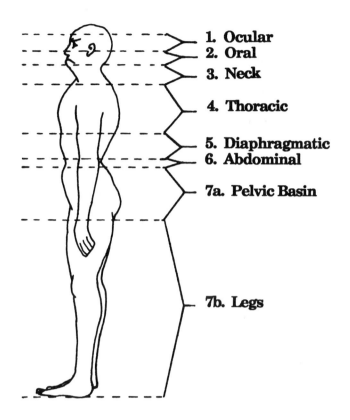

1. Ocular
2. Oral
3. Neck
4. Thoracic
5. Diaphragmatic
6. Abdominal
7a. Pelvic Basin
7b. Legs

As a natural response to pain or danger we may tighten or paralyze ourselves. Armor (overly contracted or excessively soft tissue) develops from our habitual responses, which form when we begin to anticipate a danger which is no longer really present. Armor can be looked at as physical, emotional, and mental segments which encircle the body and block its flexible and spontaneous movement. Here we see seven segments or bands of armor: 1) the ocular segment forms a defense which includes contraction, stiffness, or immobility around the scalp, forehead, eyelids, eyeballs, and tear glands and reveals a frozen, masklike or empty expression; 2) the oral segment includes the lips, chin, and throat and holds repressed needs to suck, bite, and yell; 3) the neck segment often holds back anger and swallowed feelings; 4) the thoracic segment can be stiff with controlled, pulled back shoulders or collapsed with chronic sorrow and weakness; 5) the diaphragmatic segment may cut the upper half of the person from the lower, not allowing the head and heart above, to connect with the pelvis, below; 6) the abdominal segment is around the intestines, stomach, pancreas, liver, and kidneys and holds deep gut feelings such as disgust and fear of dying; 7) the pelvic segment has two parts, 7a, the pelvic basin, which holds our deepest sexual longings and frustrations, and 7b, the legs, which hold our insecurities and lack of grounding.

SESSION I: THE UPPER HALF

BODY READING

See general notes on body reading. Share what is happening with your client's breathing. Notice that either the upper chest or diaphragmatic breathing may be neglected. Experiment with breathing in the neglected half. Also note that even when there is movement in both halves of the rib cage, there may be a block between the two which prevents a flowing, rocking breath. Share your attitude about how your client blocks feelings in breathing. Notice the position of the shoulders: whether they are pulled forward in protection, fear, or sorrow; or whether they are pulled back (and often too high) in pride or overstriving. See how the neck and chin connect with the cage and shoulders. Also share what you see with respect to the flatness of the torso: whether it is short and square -- share possibility for lengthening and rounding. This may seem simple and obvious but most people have ideals from fashion and sports, and it is important to help them understand new directions.

BODY AREA

Although this session is normally the upper half of the body, it is interchangeable with the lower half, If for some reason it is not appropriate to begin on top, begin with the legs. Also the first and second sessions can be mixed, a part being on top, a part on the bottom in each session. Normally it is important to open the breathing so that the energy can be kept at a high level for work on other areas.

1. Segments of Thoracic Cage. Generally the strategy is to begin at the bottom of the cage and work upward, the upper chest and back being released after the diaphragm and lower ribs.

    A. Diaphragmatic Band and Abdominal Mid Section. See circled numbers 1, 2, and 3 in illustrations for first session. These two bands of armor are treated together at the bottom of the rib cage where we cut off our breathing and at the middle of the abdomen where we hold in our gut feelings. Most people have contracted bands around these areas and place too much power in their exhalation and work too hard at holding in their bellies. The job is to open the abdomen-waist and lower rib cage all the way around the body and to stretch the superficial tissue under and over the diaphragmatic arch. Think of the abdomen as a balloon that opens in all directions allowing the abdominal contents to settle into the pelvis, rather than a heavy lump of organs which has to be pulled back into the abdominal cavity. Eventually this falling inside the pelvis can happen, although in the beginning (since our work is incomplete) we may even accentuate the belly falling out. Also consider the lower rib cage to be like an opening parachute or umbrella which needs to open all the way around at the bottom. A strategy for encouraging these openings is to split the sides of the rib cage spreading tissue in one direction toward the front and toward the back in the other. The chest and diaphragm nearly always need to be lifted in the front, so strokes will be upward. Also we are working across muscle structures in order to allow the musculature underneath to lengthen (as plucking across a guitar string eventually lengthens it). This work on the diaphragm will be symmetric -- some on one side some on the other, before proceeding higher on the thoracic cage.

    B. Mid-Thoracic Band. See circles 4, 5, 6 and 7 in illustrations. This band of armor prevents rocking and fluttering of the chest during breathing in the front and disorganizes the shoulder blades in the back by pulling them too far forward,

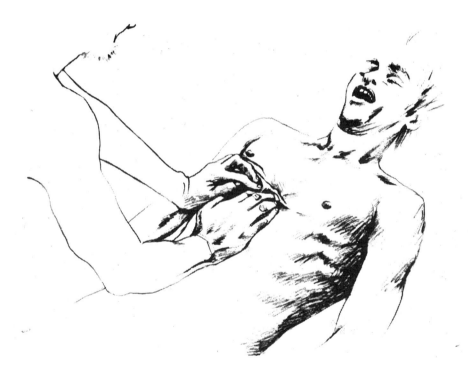

During the first phase, the practitioner hooks just beneath the surface of the skin and frees the superficial fascia, a thin envelope that stretches over the whole body, and which, when free in its function, lubricates, guides, and supports the body's mass.

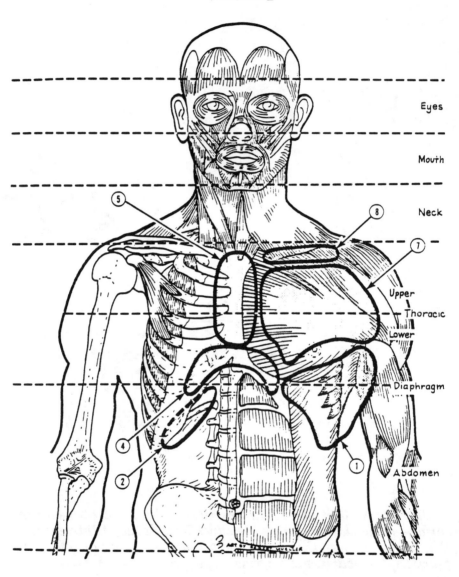

Eyes

Mouth

Neck

Upper

Thoracic

Lower

Diaphragm

Abdomen

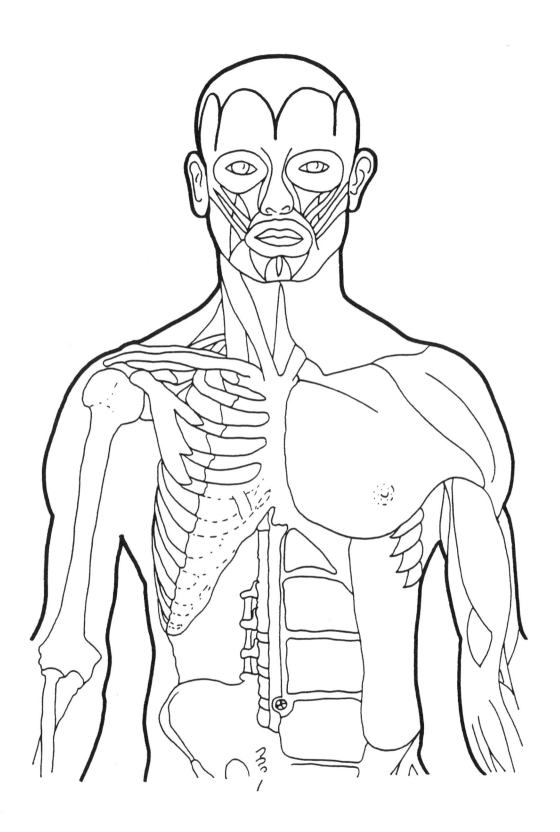

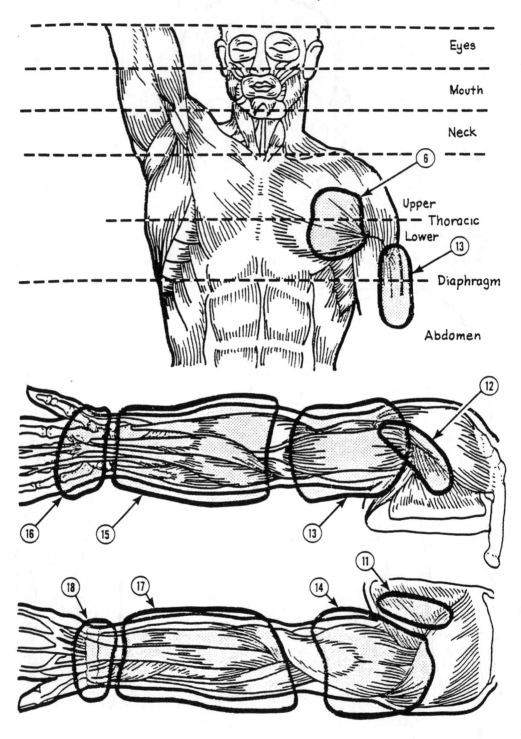

Eyes

Mouth

Neck

6

Upper
Thoracic
Lower

13

Diaphragm

Abdomen

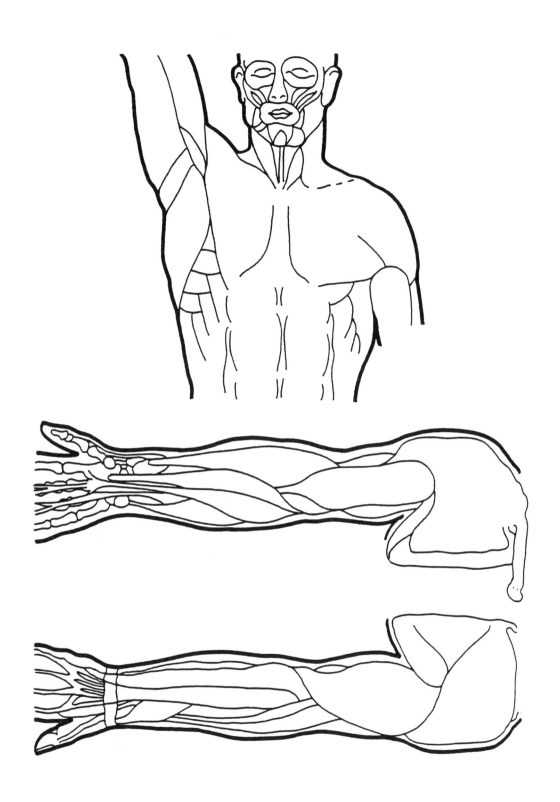

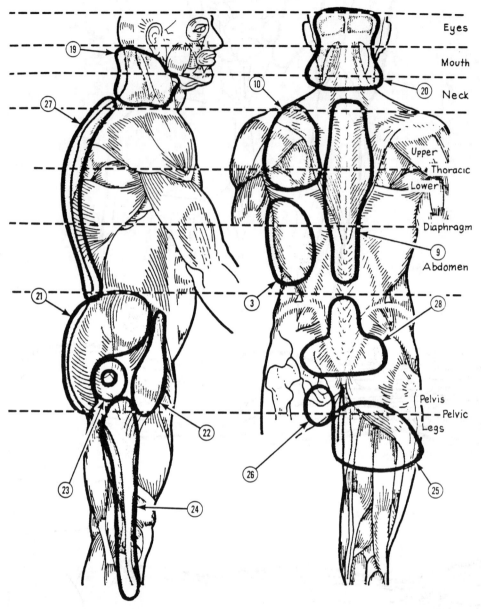

Eyes

Mouth

Neck

Upper
Thoracic
Lower

Diaphragm

Abdomen

Pelvis
Pelvic
Legs

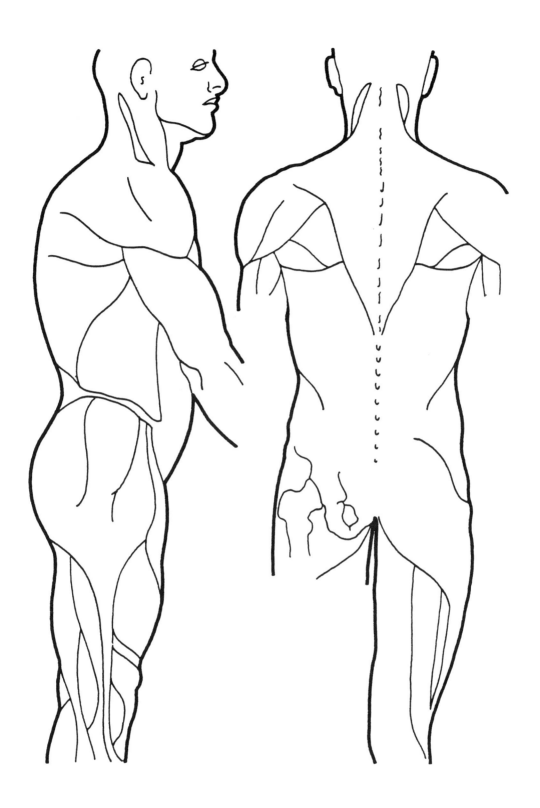

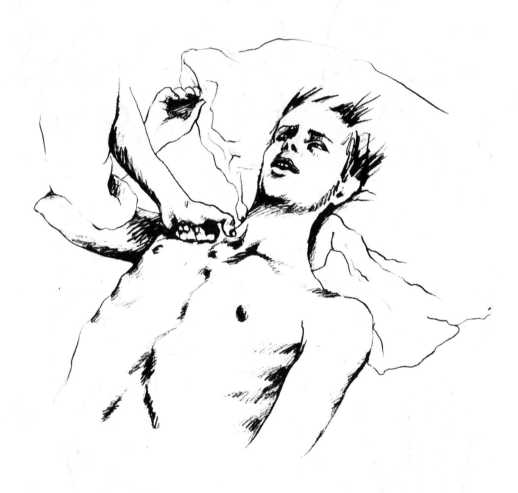

While encouraging full, free breathing, the practitioner connects myofascial planes between different parts of the body.

leaving the lower rhomboids too weak and the upper rhomboids too contracted. In the front it is important to work upward and inward in short strokes toward the breast bone. A vibrating Reichian style hand pressure on the middle of the chest, before and after tissue strokes, can help the chest collapse and expand in this central region. In the back you can use the rope-like muscles on either side of the spine (sacrospinalis) as a support for horizontally pulling the superficial tissue outward or inward (strum across these muscles). This strumming can also be rapid and provocative and can be coordinated with stimulation of the cough reflex (press on the wind pipe in front). This is not an attempt to get a full release of these deep muscles, rather they are being used as an underlying support for gripping the superficial tissue. See segment 9.

BODY READING: At this point stand your model up and look at what's happening.

C. Upper Thoracic Segment (Upper Chest, Clavicle, and Upper Trapezius as one Segment). See circles 5, 6, 7, 8, 9 and 10. In front work across the grain of the pectoralis major. Lift superficial tissue from under the clavicle, pulling it in single, sustained strokes over the bone. Same for coracoid process, pulling superficial tissue over the anterior shoulder. Here we are not working with deep fascia on the bones, but merely using the bones (tendons and ligaments) as supports for gathering and holding the superficial tissue while we stretch it. While working with the pectoralis major, use a gentle but stimulating Reichian shaking maneuver: grab both sides of the pectoralis major with the fingers underneath and thumbs on top and shake the whole body back and forth, encouraging the client to make open sounds. The same can be done with both sides of the upper trapezius, while the model is lying face down. Some slow tissue strokes may also be needed over the shoulder blades in the back and across the latissimus dorsi on the sides in order to connect the opening of this band all the way around the body (upper chest under the axilla on the sides and upper shoulder blades and trapezius on the back. Be sure to keep your provocative Reichian strokes separate from the slow, reorganization of connective tissue.

BODY READING. Stand your client up again and observe.

D. Arms As Extension of Upper Thoracic Segment. See circles 11 through 18. The superficial tissue of the upper thoracic segment cannot completely open until the arms are also released. Bioenergetic exercises which activate wanting and needing (use Crab and Jellyfish exercises) or anger (Grand Slam with tennis racket or arms) can be good before, during, or after work on the arms. It is important to connect the upper arm with the chest in front and with the shoulder blade in back. Broad, cross handed strokes can be helpful. It is important that the movement of the model's arm be precise. The shoulder is stabilized with equal contractions in the front (pectoralis major) and back (lower rhomboids). The movement of the arm comes only from the glenoid cavity without the shoulder losing its position. This is a slow movement in which the client interacts with the steady pressure of the practitioner; if you press too hard the model won't be able to move at all. Connecting the upper arm and forearm calls for similar two handed cross movements (both on the inner and outer arm) and for an interactive movement at the elbow, again without moving the shoulder. This movement is difficult for the model; take enough time to get it right. In connecting the forearm and wrist, be sure to lift tissue out of the crevice at the wrist between the ulna and radius. Work with one arm then the other.

2. Neck Segment. See circles 19 and 20. When tissue has been lifted on the chest, tension tends to shift upward into the front and eventually into the back of the neck.

Continue the work which started with lifting the superficial tissue over the clavicle, by using the fists on either side of the neck, while the head turns. (The client can be in a sitting position). Use the precise Feldenkrais exercise in which the eyes look in one direction, while the head turns in the opposite with plenty of distance between the ear lobes and shoulder tips. Also work along the occiput, across the capitis muscles, to lengthen the back of the neck (either with knuckles from the side of neck or with finger tips while model is lying on back). This is important: to equalize the lengthening of the anterior chest with the lengthening of the posterior neck. This lengthening of the posterior neck can also be coordinated with work over the top of the trapezius. Have your model sit on a chair or on the knees and with the flat part of your elbow pull the superficial tissue from the anterior superior part of the trapezius, over the bulk of the muscle backward and then downward to the shoulder blades. The model needs to maintain an upright symmetric position. As you execute these moves, have your client imagine a milk maid's wooden collar with buckets of milk on either end stabilizing and lowering the shoulders.

BODY READING: Look at what's happened to this point.

3. Pelvic Segment. (If there is not enough time, this segment can be done during the second session). See circles 21 through 28. This area, around the pelvis and on the outer surface of the iliotibial tract, is important for balancing the changes which occur in the thoracic segment with the lower half of the body. (It can be done before the neck segment). If, after opening the thoracic area, we were not eventually to work with the pelvic segment, the upper half of the body would lift forward, pulling the lower posterior half with it, and exaggerating any lordosis and not allowing the diaphragmatic breathing to be complete in the back, where it needs to connect with the sacrum and hips.

> **A. Around the Greater Trochanter.** Split the tissue above the trochanter by first working backward and downward over the gluteus maximus. The fists or flats of the elbows will be helpful with this often dense and resistant tissue. Have your client use the pelvic curl as an interacting movement. Then, while still above the trochan ter, use the knuckles, or slightly sharper elbow to hook the superficial tissue, just behind the tensor fascia lata, and push the tissue in an anterior-superior direction over the muscle. Careful, this area calls for balance, force, and calm and can be painful for the model, but don't worry, the structure is not fragile. Client abducts thigh and rotates medially.

> **B. Iliotibial Tract.** The client lies on side, a pillow between the legs, to preserve parallel lines between legs. This area has much to do with whether the hip and knee can function together in a forward straight line. Our earliest feelings, as we learn to walk (confidence, fear, insecurity), are locked into this hard string, which guides the upper leg. Use a double stroke, one flat elbow above, another below, zigzagging along the tract. Careful at the bottom of the tract not to bunch the tissue at the lateral knee. You can use extra strokes to stretch the tissue toward the front and back of the upper leg on either side of the tract.

> **C. Ischial Release.** (This work can also be done in the second session). With the client on the back, knees bent, have the client pull one knee straight toward the chest. (Be sure to respect the parallel body lines). Work across the tissue just inferior to the ischium on one (bent) side; then pull the tissue across the middle of the ischium. Finally reach inside to the medial, flat surface of the ischium and pull the tissue out and over the surface of the ischium. You can use the fingers to reach this inner area, while clamping with the thumb on the outside. It's really important for the whole body structure that the ischia are not too narrow in their

distance from one another. If they are too close together, there will not be a sufficient arch (across the pelvis), as in a cathedral, to support easily the above weight, and stress will be thrown into the hips and knees. Many women have excessive flesh around the hips because their ischia are too close together. Clearly there is a great deal of sexual significance to this area as well.

D. Pelvic Curl. Take time to begin teaching the use of the psoas. Use your fingertips under a flat back, during a pelvic curl, to stretch the lumbar fascia, while the psoas is activated and belly is relaxed. The client may need this work in every session to learn finally what's happening.

4. Final Neck Movement. See circle 19. Repeat the stroke diagonal across the neck with the eyes looking at the opposite shoulder, while the head turns. This is used at the end of every session to rebalance the neck in relation to the changes that have taken place during the session.

5. Spinal Roll. See circle 27. From a kneeling position or while sitting on a chair (shoulders stabilized), have the model roll forward one vertebra at a time, while you slowly zigzag with your elbows down the side of the spine, pulling superficial tissue over the sacrospinalis. Let this be a gentle roll. Pressing too hard will require too much resistance from your client. Use your fists (both simultaneously) to complete the lower back and sacrum.

FINAL BODY READING

Help your client feel the difference in the range of breathing by holding your hands on chest, belly, and diaphragm. Use a mirror to point out the changes in shape: higher upper chest, rounder in the cage, etc.

FINAL FINE ENERGY

Be sure to save time at the end of the session for this work. Brush meridians, and use points to harmonize the energy flow. But if there is unfinished business, work with this, before regulating fine energy. Bring some energy back down into the legs, where there has been little work, so that the client can rediscover his or her grounding. During the session it is important, from time to time, to do some energy work on the lower part of the body, so that it will not be too neglected. You can use images to help harmonize the energy.

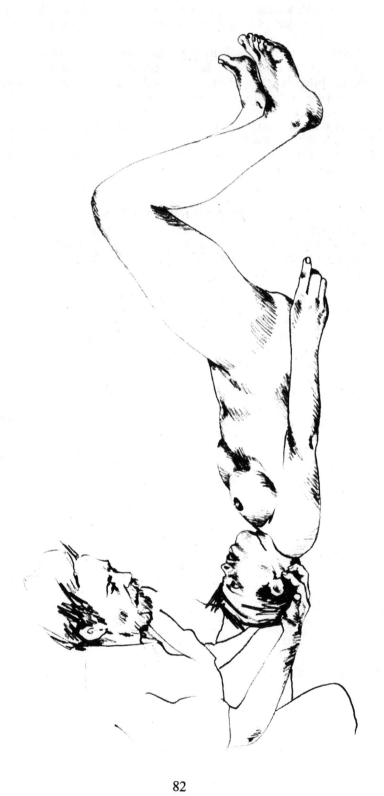

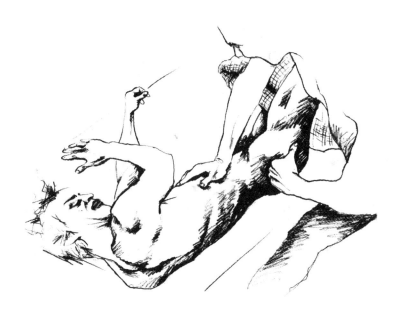

SESSION 2: THE LOWER HALF

BODY READING

See general notes on bodyreading in Part I. Notice that the foot has three arches (medial, transverse and lateral). The weight of the body can be evenly distributed through these three. In the case of a weak medial arch (flat feet) note how the excessive eversion places tension on the lateral arch and the tissue around the fibula. The shaft of the fibula may be rotated and shifted too far forward. Notice in the case of an overly arched medial arch that the tension is on the inner lower leg, lifting the arch inward and upward. At the same time the transverse arch may be also too high and narrow. Notice the connection between these arches and what happens in the rest of the body, e.g., flat feet and knock knees, high medial arches and bow legs. Help your clients experience their structural tendencies and alternatives. Look at what's happening with dorsi-flexion and plantar flexion. Women who wear high heels will be excessively plantar flexed with a shortened achilles tendon. (Even normal men's heels will have some effect in this direction). On the other hand, look at the excessive dorsi flexion involved in cases where the weight is mostly on the heels. Note that shoes with negative heels and built in arches are eventually counterproductive, since these artificial positions will produce compensatory tensions in other parts of the structure. The foot needs a natural, broad last, and an even (flat) and soft sole.

BODY AREA

The general aim is to bring together the sections of superficial fascia: fascia pedis, plantar fascia, fascia cruris. This gives space for the toes, ankles, and knees to begin working more together. Also this opening of tissue from the feet upward into the legs need to be connected with the work already started on the fascia lata (envelope around the whole thigh) by work around and above the knee and with the hamstrings as far upward as the ischium. Before beginning, you may want to use some of these exercises: Marching, Snap Kick, ...

1. Fascia Pedis (top of foot). See circled number 1. Imagine old fashion spats or anklets covering the top of the foot. We want to expand them all the way around the foot and ankle. With the client on the back, begin on the front and work across the tendons of the toes, while interacting with toe movements. Continue around the sides of the foot, crossing the tendons of the tibialis anterior on one side, and the peroneals, on the other. Let this work go all the way back to the achilles tendon. Remember we are not trying to work on deep fascia, but are using the underlying structures to help us get hold of the superficial tissue. One common problem is gripping (or in the extreme, hammer) toes. Note that the tension is not only on the top of the foot, but also underneath, in the plantar fascia. Try to hook the top and bottom of the toes at the same time (with thumb on top and first knuckle on the bottom), and pull toward the end of the toe.

2. Connecting Fascia Pedis with:

A. Anterior Cruris (Front of lower leg). See circled numbers 2 and 3. Work across the front of the ankle. Pull tissue across these large tendons, while the ankle moves (in alignment with the knee). To get hold of the tissue you may need to use relatively sharp knuckles, inserted between the internal and external malleolus. Continue upward, going in between the tibia and the tibialis anterior, across the tibialis anterior, digitorum and peroneous (outward toward the fibula). Separately, or simultaneously, you may work across the tibia, across the flat part

84

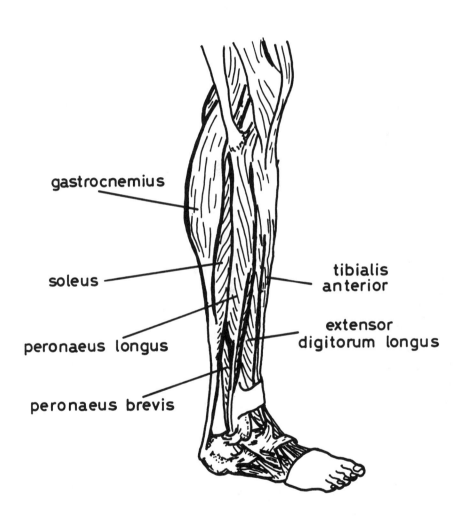

gastrocnemius

soleus

peronaeus longus

peronaeus brevis

tibialis
anterior

extensor
digitorum longus

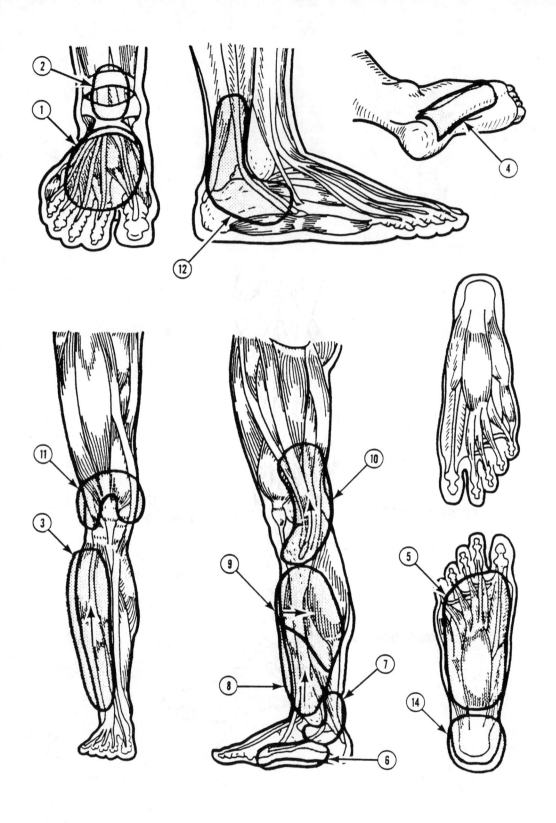

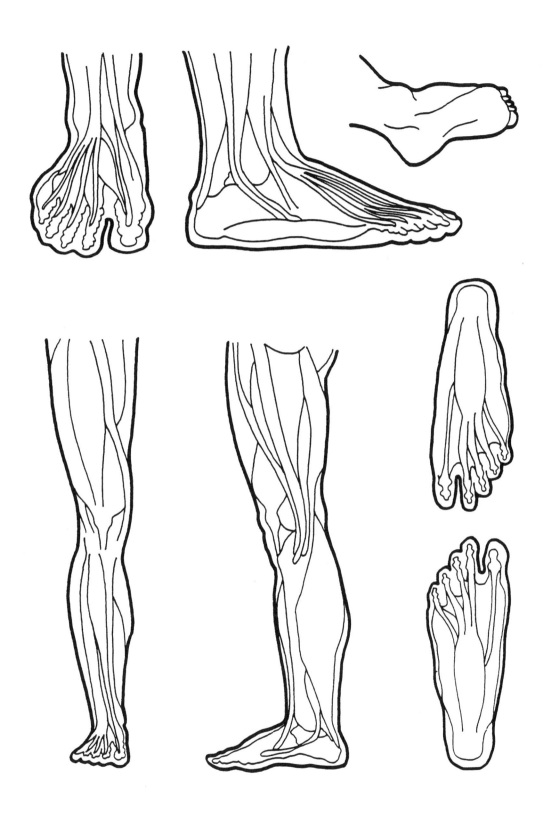

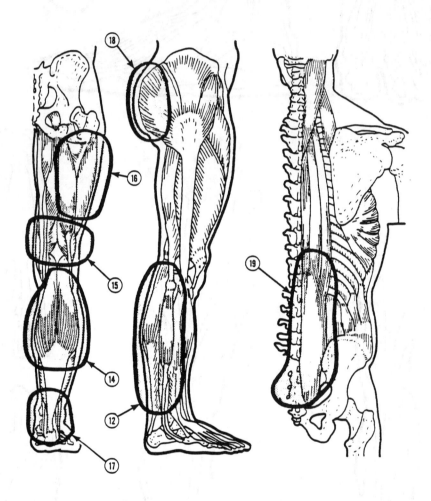

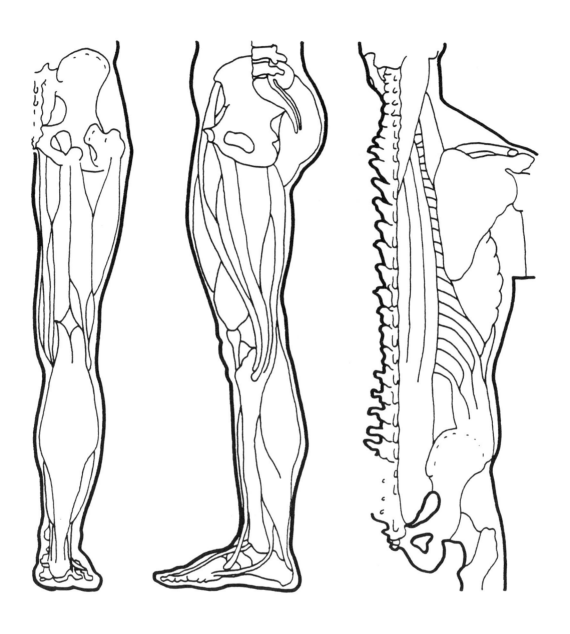

of the shin. Working in these two opposite directions opens the fascia cruris in the front of the lower leg. Here your client may encounter pains and memories from old injuries. We have all banged our legs a lot, sometimes so painfully that we have repressed the experience completely.

B. Plantar Fascia (bottom of foot). See circled numbers 4 through 6. The sole of the foot can be broadened by using the heels of the hands on top for reinforcement, and the fingers underneath to spread the ball outward in all directions. Lift the foot and bend the knee. Now you can use your knuckles on the sole of the heel. You can also work, simultaneously, on the bottom and top of the foot -- the knuckles of one hand raking underneath, while the heel of the other hand works diagonally across the tendons on top. Spreading of the plantar area allows other connections above, and also allows the weight of the foot to be more evenly distributed. After working on the foot, have the model stand and feel the possibility of having a broad foot which spreads in all directions. Do this again after you've worked on the whole leg.

C. Medial Cruris (medial lower leg). See circles 7 and 8. Have your client on the side with a pillow to keep parallelism between the legs. Connect the medial foot with medial lower leg, while the ankle moves -- use of a two handed cross movement working across tibialis posterior, soleus, and gastrocnemius. Continue hooking along and across these muscles. One possibility is to use the broad, flat part of both fists at the same time, raking the whole sheath (medial cruris from the tibia to the full part of the gastrocnemius).

D. Lateral Cruris (lateral lower leg around fibula). See circles 11 and 12. Have the client sit side saddle, giving an even, flat support to both the ankle and knee. While the model moves the ankle, use two handed strokes to connect the lateral foot and the tissue on either side of the fibula. Continue along the lower lateral leg, dividing tissue outward (anterior and posterior), away from the fibula (over the peroneals), while the client continues to move the ankle.

3. Connecting Fascia Cruris with Fascia Lata (whole thigh).

A. With the client lying on the side, as in medial lower leg work, now use a two handed cross stroke to connect the tissue of the medial lower leg with the tissue of the medial thigh. See circle 9. One hand will work just above the knee (across·the confluence of the semitendinosus, semimembranosus, gracilis, and sartorius). Now the client's movement is at both the ankle and knee at the same time. Keep these strokes broad and superficial. The action of the client will help create a stretch between the lower and upper legs.

B. Client is in side saddle position. Connect the lateral lower leg with the tissue worked in the first session (iliotibial tract) with a two handed stroked across the knee. Now the client moves both the ankle and knee, with the knee movement beginning at the ankle. (Consult movement awareness exercises in Chapter V).

C. Use fingers or knuckles, while client is in same position, to work around the front of the knee, beginning at the bottom of the knee, and going upward, along the sides, and pincering together, under and over the rectus femoris, above the knee. The action is in ankle and knee. See circle 10.

D. With client on back, knees bent, and movement coming from the ankle, grip hands from front of knee around to popliteal fossa. Your hands pull outward across the tendons behind knees, while the knee moves. The heels of hands support the hands in front. See circle 15.

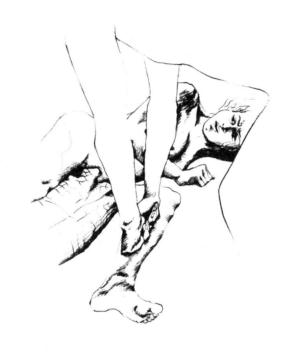

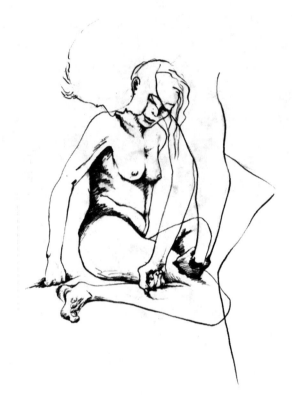

E. Do the same for the gastrocnemius, grabbing between its two parts and separating them as the foot dorsi and plantar flexes. See circle 14.

F. Hold the foot in maximum dorsi flexion and with the knuckles of both hands pull on either side of the achilles tendon all the way to the calcaneous. Client stretches tendon. See circle 17.

4. Connecting Posterior Fascia Lata (hamstrings) with Ischia and Buttocks. While your client is on belly and straightens and relaxes arms, spread the tissue inward and outward across both groups of hamstrings. With one hand work outward across biceps femoris while with the other stretch over the ischium -- across biceps but across gluteal fascia. It is important to create plenty of length all along the back of the legs, and the back of the pelvis. This helps connect the lower posterior body to diaphragmatic breathing. See circles 16 and 18.

5. Neck and Spinal Roll (as in first session).

FINAL FINE ENERGY

Again, as in the first session, take enough time to harmonize the parts you have already worked (lower half), with the unattended part (upper half). Help the client understand how good grounding supports and frees the upper part of the body.

PHASE II: ELONGATION

(Session 3)

GENERAL PURPOSE

We now want to loosen an intermediate layer of tissue between the pelvis, rib cage, and shoulders, mostly along the lateral torso. This is an elongation of Bodymind along the sides, from hips to shoulders. This lengthening gives space for the pelvis and rib cage to move more freely, independent of each other (quadratus lumborum must lengthen). It also begins the rounding of the rib cage and lifting of the 11th and 12th ribs, giving more space for posterior inhalation. Draw an imaginary line along the center of the side of the body, and divide the tissue forward and backward along this line so that the hips widen from front to back, the rib cage expands in both directions, and the shoulders settle into a central position, with the pectoralis muscles relaxing in the front and the trapezius and rhomboids in the back. Also work for a balance between the medial (latissimus dorsi, and teres major) and lateral (teres minor, infraspinatus) rotators of the arm. We are looking for a three dimensional expansions of the person as opposed to the feeling of being a front or back, or having sides. We need fullness and flexibility throughout the whole torso. Review the artifacts of classical Greek sculpture. Read Rilke's poem on viewing Venus de Milo.

BODY TYPE

1.   **Squat, short torso types** whose length has been arrested during adolescence, need lots of deep work between the crest of the ilium and the twelfth rib. Many men have inflated chests but short torsos.

2.   **Long waisted types** (many women) potentially have a great deal of flexibility but may protect themselves from what they consider excessive sensuality by tightening the sacrospinalis. The work on the latissimus dorsi should extend all the way around the torso to the spine and the sacrospinalis.

3. **Burdened and Needy types** may need plenty of work on the pectoralis minor in order to allow the shoulders to shift posterior. And Rigid types may need more loosening between the shoulder blades for the shoulders to shift forward.

EMOTION

In contrast with the first phase, some deeper emotions may begin to surface, but generally clients will not completely confront their deepest problems. Most of the session is along the sides of the torso and back, and will often evoke feelings of fear and vulnerability. You may also encounter sexual fear, which blocks the flowing, swinging interaction between the hips and ribs. Also the arms may be pulled around toward the front to protect the sexual organs. Going beyond these fears, of course, we can encourage the confidence of an open chest, and the sensuality of a flowing mid-body.

The sides of the body connect with the arms and help govern their position and rotation. We may hold our arms and shoulders back, rotating them out in readiness or we may hold our arms in front, rotating them inward in protection. A lot of wanting and holding back are in the arms.

THOUGHT AND AFFIRMATION

Our image of ourselves often involves just the front of the body, and when we begin to feel ourselves all the way around the torso, we begin to think of our environment less as something to be confronted and more of a space in which we expand simultaneously in all

95

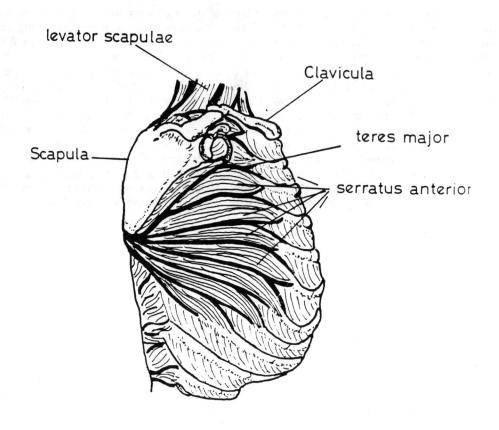

levator scapulae

Clavicula

teres major

Scapula

serratus anterior

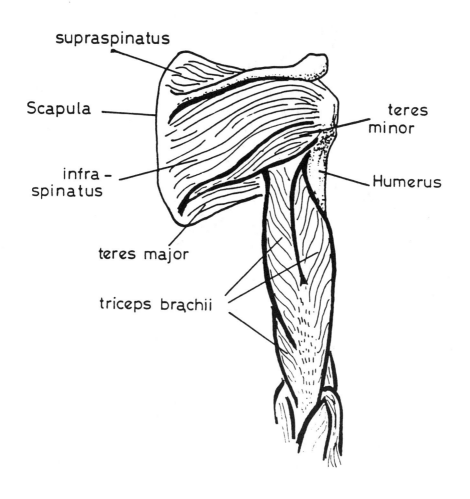

supraspinatus

Scapula

infra-
spinatus

teres major

triceps brachii

teres
minor

Humerus

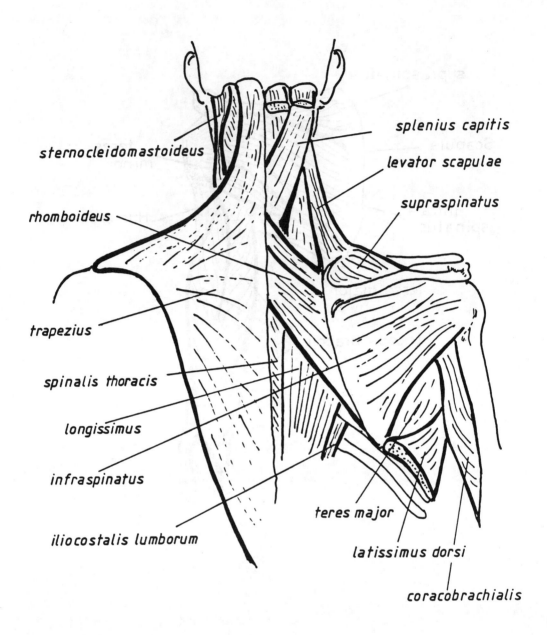

sternocleidomastoideus

splenius capitis

levator scapulae

supraspinatus

rhomboideus

trapezius

spinalis thoracis

longissimus

infraspinatus

teres major

latissimus dorsi

iliocostalis lumborum

coracobrachialis

directions. "I claim the space behind me as well as what's in front of me." "I am I and all that's around me." (cf Ortega y Gasset). Also "I can be long, supple and sensual, while at the same time being proud and strong." "I have a long waist and I expand my rib cage."

MANIPULATIONS

1. **Depth, Speed, Distance.** The angle of entry is steeper, going through the superficial layer of tissue and beginning the work on the tops of the individual envelopes. This is not the deepest work, which will penetrate to attachments, but does begin to separate and lengthen muscles. After reaching an appropriate depth, it is now important to go much slower, to wait for the deeper tissue to open, and finally, to move a shorter distance. If these strokes are well executed, you will need to cover less area than in the first phase, since any deep release will have an extensive effect in other parts of the body.

2. **Since the work is not as broad** as in the first phase, the points of the elbow or the knuckles, will be useful in contrast with the flat parts of the fist, or sides or backs of the hand, as used in the first sessions. Also two-handed two-directional work will be less frequent, since we are concentrating more on depth.

3. **Lots of participation** is needed from the client in order to get the tissue in deep, relatively inaccessible areas to move and change. For example, when working on the pectoralis minor, be sure the client moves downward and forward at the shoulder; and when sliding into the anterior part of the scapula, have your client move both arms upward until the hands touch; or when reaching the subscapularis from behind, have your client hold the arm behind the back and then flex the rhomboids, while you slide under the scapula.

BREATH AND ENERGY WORK

Focus less on exploring charge and discharge and more now on ways of sustaining energy. Use the connected and sustained breath techniques to maintain an even emotional and energy level, during what may be painful manipulations. We are working deeper and need to encourage the model to begin to sort out feelings and to stay with one feeling at a time -- all of which calls for a sustained level of energy. Encourage breathing in the posterior rib cage (using images, and a light, guiding touch). Some helpful exercises are The Crab, Picking Fruit, The Grand Slam.

MOVEMENT AWARENESS

While interacting with your strokes, the client needs now to move carefully only certain muscles. We want to separate and isolate muscles from their neighbors. But the focus is still on extrinsic muscles, the large powerful muscles of locomotion. Half way through the third session, have the client experiment with arm, shoulder and torso movements, comparing the released side with the untouched side. Most people don't want to explore how far back they can move their arms and shoulders and will need a lot of encouragement and support to discover that such stiff, unconscious areas can come to life again.

MERIDIANS AND POINTS

The gall bladder and spleen meridians are important to this session. Underneath the fear we feel along the sides and back is expanding yang anger which can be released by scratching and slapping along the gall bladder meridian. Also the top of the shoulder is another important retainer of gall bladder anger. Important points: Gb 25, 29, 30, also gall bladder points along the temples, Sp 21, Liv 14, Doors of Life (Gv 4, B23, B47).

CHAKRAS

This phase helps connect the navel, heart and throat chakras.

SESSION 3

(Lateral Torso)

BODYREADING

Look at the imaginary line along the side of the body to see if excessive tension is more in the front or back of the body. From front and back, look at whether one side of the waist is more contracted than the other. What is the relation of this tension, on one side of the waist, to other tensions in the shoulder, on the opposite side, or to adduction of the leg also on the other side? Help your client trace and feel these interconnections. Do the arms rotate inward or outward? Are the shoulders pulled forward or back? Remember there can be lots of fear in the cage and shoulders.

BODY AREAS

Except where indicated, this work is all done with the client lying on the side, the legs made parallel with a support (cushion).

1. Pelvic Segment (Intermediate). See circled number 1. This is a reworking of the same area as in session one, except we are working now with the envelopes of the gluteus maximus and tensor fascia lata. This deeper release will allow more expansion on both sides of the cage and help provide space for the release of the quadratus lumborum. Don't be afraid to go fairly deep with your elbow.

2. Lower and middle Segments of Thoracic Cage. See circled numbers 3 and 4. Now we are working along the segments where we also worked in session one but are specifically pulling backward across the latissimus dorsi (while the client rotates the arm inward) and pulling forward over the serratus anterior muscles (during deep inhalations in the chest). Work again under the diaphragmatic arch, this time going further underneath in the direction of the attachments of the diaphragm.

3. Quadratus Lumborum. See circled number 5. We work below and above, before attempting to release the quadratus lumborum with elbow, knuckles, or reinforced finger tips. Be careful not to press directly against the floating ribs. Have your client make a hip movement to the side, to activate the quadratus lumborum. At this point you should begin to see a fuller expansion of diaphragmatic breathing with the inhalations rippling down into the hips.

4. Upper Segment of Thoracic Cage. See circled numbers 6 through 10. (Client is lying on side). Here we are working below the axilla and under the pectoralis major toward the front and arm rotators toward the back, along the shoulder blade. Don't work directly in the axilla, but slide the fingertips under the latissimus dorsi, while the client rotates the arm medially. In front slide your fingertips under the pectoralis major, while the client moves the shoulder forward and back again. While the client is on the back, we can also work directly on the pectoralis minor (circle 12) by penetrating through the major near the coracoid process. On the shoulder blade work with the teres minor and infraspinatus, while the model rotates the arm laterally.

5. Top of shoulder and Deltoid. See circled no. 10 and 11. While the client is still on the side work along the top of the shoulder, deep in the supraspinatus with the knuckles while your client lifts the arm as in a flying movement. Further along the

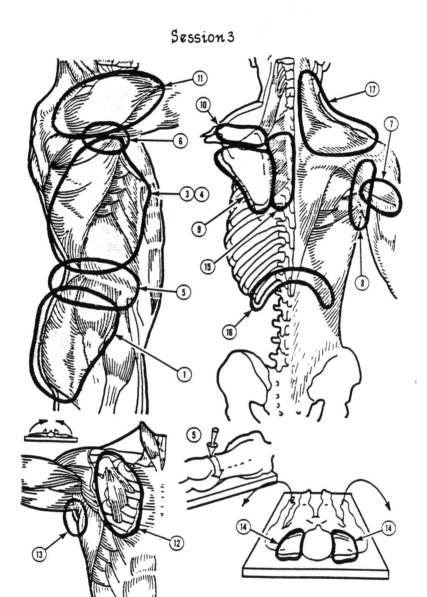

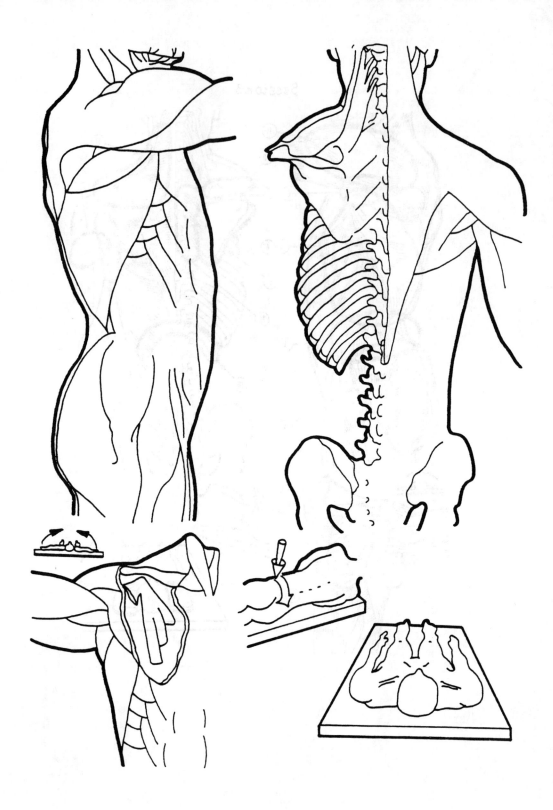

top of the shoulder toward the neck and around the medial portion of the shoulder blade, the shoulder is lifted (levator scapula and trapezius). Now go directly to the middle fibers of the deltoid, and use the flying motion of the arm again. In the lateral and medial fibers of the deltoid use forward flexion and backward extension of the whole upper arm. The client's deltoid can be very hard (especially in body workers) and these fibers, which do different jobs, need to be separated. The front, back, top, and tip of the shoulder will begin to soften and balance with each other. You can give your client the image of a milkmaid's yoke to help lower and stabilize the shoulder, and separate arm movements from shoulder movements.

HALF WAY READING

Have your model stand up, and now compare one side with the other. Be sure you have a large full length mirror. Take time to point out the exact changes.

SECOND HALF

Follow the above procedure of working with body areas on the other half of the body.

SYMMETRIC WORK

After work is complete on both sides of the body, there are some other possible areas for work, on both sides of the body.

1. 11th and 12th Ribs. See circled number 16. With your model on the belly, use your fingertips and the thumbs of both hands to lift up, over and in between, the 12th and then the 11th ribs. This movement encourages the rounding and opening of diaphragmatic breathing, as well as indirectly influencing the upper thoracic structures. The movement must be slow and precise, and be done sufficiently under the ribs.

2. First Rib. See circle 14. Now go to the other end of the rib cage and with the client on the back press your fingertips into the thoracic inlet and onto the first rib. Deep breathing and arm movements can help your client interact with your strokes. Another interacting movement is for the client to lift the arms from the sides of the body upward, in front, to shoulder level. The first rib is often immobile, like a frozen lock on the top of the rib cage. Together with the mobility of the 11th and 12th ribs, the free movement of the first rib can have a rippling effect throughout the whole rib cage.

3. Subscapularis. See circle 13. With fingertips, work under the shoulder blade from the front, while your client is on back. The arms are brought together with slight rotations. Careful, this can be very painful. This work is especially needed when adduction and medial rotation of the arm is too great and the shoulder blades are pulled too far forward.

4. Over The Top of the Shoulders. See circle 17. While the client is seated, use the flat part of the elbow to rake from the front of the shoulders diagonal back across the top of the shoulders and shoulder blades. Be sure the client maintains a good position with the shoulder stabilized, chin in, and neck flat. The client can assist by holding the head slightly down and rotating the head.

5. Neck and Back. Usual strokes across neck and down the back.

103

FINAL FINE ENERGY

Work with the feeling of wholeness and roundness. While your model is sitting or standing, brush the yin and yang meridians of the front and back (or sides) simultaneously. The image of expanding in all directions, inside a sphere, helps develop a more complete spacial feeling.

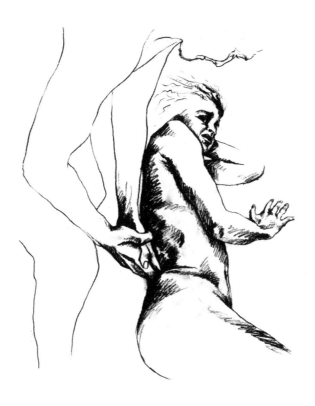

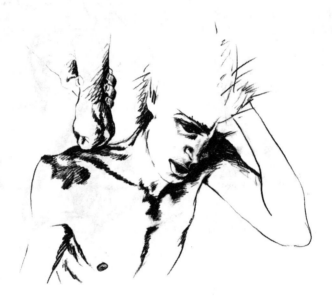

PHASE III: PELVIC RELEASE

(Sessions 4, 5, and 6)

GENERAL PURPOSE

We now want to release deep armor on the bottom, top, and back of the pelvis. We are unravelling the third level of fascia which wraps around the underside of muscles, and extends to the attachments on the periosteum. By freeing the pelvis from forward or backward imbalances, sideway tilts, and clockwise or counterclockwise twists, we help bring the head, above, and the legs, below, into a more efficient alignment and give the spine a chance to straighten itself. The floor of the pelvis can begin to move like a diaphragm, contracting evenly up and down, in coordination with the breathing diaphragm. This movement of the pelvic floor (pubococcygeus) enlivens sexual response and satisfaction. The release of pelvic energy, not only makes the pelvis more alive and mobile but infuses the whole body with the vitality which has been held back because of fear and guilt.

BODYTYPE

1. Anal types may be either very tense around the anus, tucking the tail under, or so open that they expose their asses. We are dealing with a holding in of rage against authority, which can easily turn into sadistic or masochistic tendencies. You can satisfy this need for pain (initially this might create satisfaction and trust) but eventually you will need to go further, dealing with the deep need for contact and stimulation; or you can work very gently and softly, refusing to accommodate the demand for pain, showing that feeling and pleasure is possible without extreme pain.

2. When there is an extreme accumulation of tension and energy around the genitalia, we may be dealing with phallic narcissism, where the penis is used as a weapon against the parents. "You excited me but didn't satisfy me, now I'm going to get even with you," or with hysteria: "I want you and need you so badly that I shudder all over." Work as above: either exhaust your client and then work gently, or keep the energy slow but aware.

3. Oral (needy) types, in concentrating their energy around the mouth and throat, these individuals may take energy away from the anus and genitals. Sometimes helping them to satisfy their oral needs (e.g., sucking their thumbs) will help them begin to pay more attention to the neglected parts of the pelvis.

4. Hysterical types can be considered a variation of oral types. The search for the love of the denied parent, contributes to an overeagerness to climax, to be completely satisfied. They are overexcited by having almost any part of the body touched but are never satisfied. Two paths: one is to stimulate them so much that they become exhausted (this takes patience), the other is to show that you still love them, even if you say no to their demands. Work with the heart chakra.

EMOTION

The pelvis often holds the deepest and most hidden emotions of the whole body. When they begin to be released, they need a channel for expression. For this reason it is important during these sessions of pelvic work to also work frequently around the eyes, in the nose, inside the mouth, with the throat and gut, in order to keep a channel open to the throat and head. If these deep pelvic feelings come to consciousness, after having been

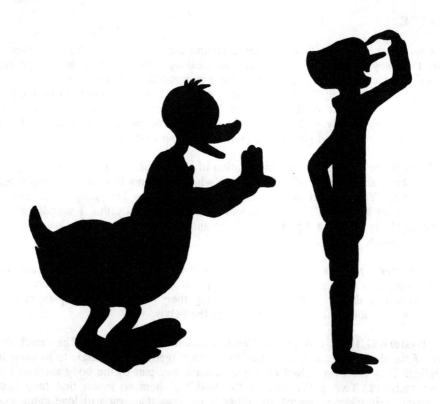

Donald Duck and Pinocchio show us how the orientation of the pelvis determines character. Donald, with tilted pelvis, arched back and splayed feet, is angry and stuck. Pinocchio, whose pelvis supports and organizes his whole structure, is open to change.

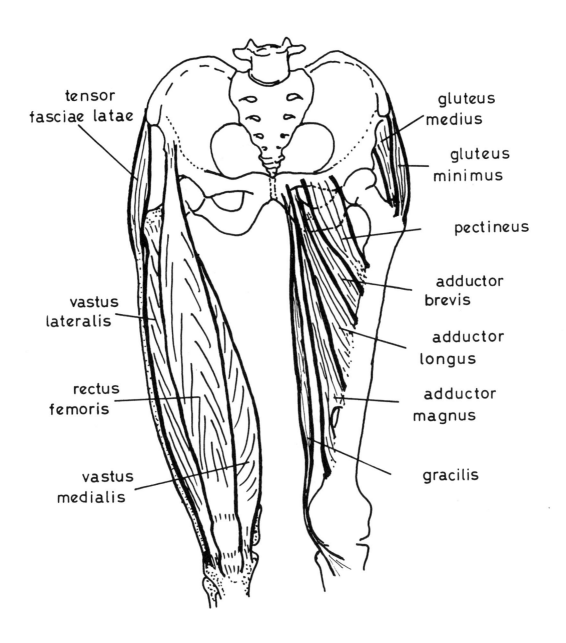

tensor
fasciae latae

gluteus
medius

gluteus
minimus

pectineus

vastus
lateralis

adductor
brevis

adductor
longus

rectus
femoris

adductor
magnus

vastus
medialis

gracilis

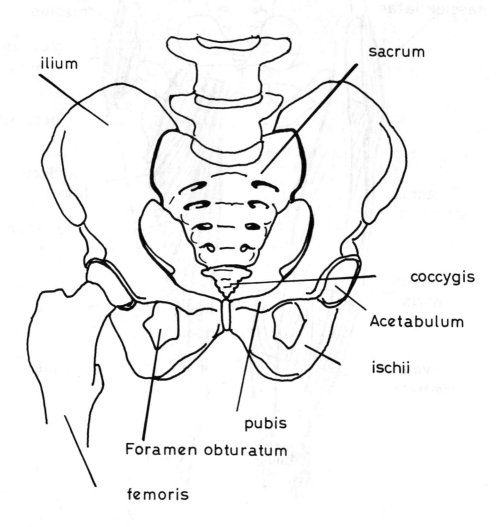

ilium

sacrum

coccygis

Acetabulum

ischii

pubis

Foramen obturatum

femoris

buried so long, but can't escape their chronic armor, uncontrollable elation and depression, nervousness, etc. may follow. Don't leave your client with this kind of unfinished business.

THOUGHT AND AFFIRMATION

The pelvis is often taboo or receives too much attention. When we begin to accept our anal and genital functions as no more important than other functions of our body, we are beginning to allow our energy to distribute more equally throughout bodymind. We can then say, "Every part of me gives me pleasure," "When I have genital energy I have it; when I don't, I don't." (Variation from EST: "When you're hot you're hot, when you're not, you're not"). Also: "I can enjoy the valleys as well as the peaks of pleasure," "Ejaculatory orgasm is great, and is not necessary for completeness."

MANIPULATIONS

1. We are now reaching for the deepest layers of tissue and our movements need to be super slow. We enter and wait for the tissue to accept our pressure at a deeper level.

2. We are now reaching for the deepest layer of tissue and need to use finger and elbow points (sharper parts) to slide in between and under muscles reaching attachments on the bone.

3. Slight weaving movements with our hands or elbows can help to probe deeper through resistant layers.

4. Slight twisting or lifting moves are appropriate after the final depth has been reached.

5. Also strumming diagonally across the muscles, especially the attachments will help lengthen their structures. Although in deep work, we are frequently sliding between muscles, separating them one from another, as we reach the deepest level, diagonal strokes (whether twisting, lifting, or strumming) are finally even more important. These deep manipulations are to be coordinated with subtle movements initiated by the client.

BREATH AND ENERGY WORK

1. When there is overeagerness and overexcitement locked in the pelvis it may be helpful to let this charge exhaust itself (with lots of fast breathing, pelvic gyrations, expressions of deep seated pelvic anger, hard fucking movements, masochistic clamping down in the ass hole) before turning to a softer style, helping the individual equalize this charge through the entire body. At this point gentle touching of the erogenous zones (genitals, anus, nipples, lips, roof of the mouth, inside the ears), while verbally discouraging rapid overcharge, can help establish a fine streaming.

2. In cases of deadness, unconsciousness, inability to sustain a charge in the pelvic area, begin slowly and spend a great deal of time building energy without losing it. Support and trust are important in getting this charge to happen. Eventually advanced work in the pelvis (Master PI) may be needed to activate an extreme lack of energy. Use the "connected and sustained breaths" (see Jack's book, Deep Bodywork and Personal Development) frequently, in order to keep the energy high. Maintain a constant charge. Don't allow your client to drift away. Direct eye contact with verbal approval and support can help overcome the negative pelvic controls, coming from mommy, daddy, and society.

3. When the individual has begun to overcome sexual taboos, encourage them to suck their thumbs, fondle their genitals and anus. These are natural parts of the body and need not have an excessive charge or be neglected, energyless parts of the self.

4. Some helpful exercises are: The Crab, Jellyfish, Spread Eagle, Barking Dog, Pelvic Drop, Pelvic Curl, Sucking, Face Stimulation, Rock and Roll, Sexual Surrender, Bottom Rub.

MOVEMENT AWARENESS

1. Using the pelvic curl (with inhalation and contraction of the psoas during upward movement), is a way of raising sexual energy and also working with fine energy at the end of the session. Let the upward curl be very slight, anything greater will involve the abdominus rectus, which should remain relaxed. Persons who want to uncurl too far (into an overarched back, lordosis) often are exhaling too much, overworking the extrinsic muscles around the diaphragm, as well as the muscles of the back. Show them that when they drop the pelvis, the exhalation does not have to continue, does not have to be forced out.

2. Curling up on the exhalation rather than on the inhalation, is the way that most people move; you can make use of this when they need to focus on discharging an access of accumulated energy. But the above movement should also eventually be explored.
3. During streaming, the pelvis will spontaneously rock in many directions, without one using either of the above exercises. The exercises are only a preparation, an exploration of possible movements.

4. Have your client press the knees (bent) outward, against your hands, then quickly change: the pressure is inward against your hands (or forearm). This changing resistance between the abductors and adductors activates lots of feeling. Try the same thing, but very gently, until there is a fine quivering throughout the legs.

5. After a session have your client walk around the room, exploring different pelvic and hip movements along with a variety of feelings and attitudes. Suggest movements which are confident beautiful, graceful, etc.

6. Instruct your clients in internal pelvic exercises, so that they may gradually gain control over the floor of the pelvis. An inner, slow lifting of the genitals and anus, and then slow release should be practiced everyday, until awareness and control of the pelvic floor is easy and complete.

MERIDIANS AND POINTS

Stomach 30, The doors of LIfe (GV 4, B23, B47). Liver 10, 11 and 12, Spleen 6, Conception Vessel 1 are all powerful points for opening or calming (self-regulating) pelvic energy. Try also combining these points with points around the head, in order to balance pelvic and head energy.

CHAKRAS

Phase III is work with the first and second chakras. Before going to higher chakras, it is important to help your clients with grounding, with accepting their sexual energy. Try some tantric exercises such as "Closing The Lover Gates," in which the genitals and anus are blocked with the hands, while the individual breathes gently upward. Try, at the same time, closing the upper gates: hands over mouth and eyes, fingers over the ears. The individual can then go into an inner meditative space. Try also having your client draw the anus upward, while an inflated diaphragm presses down against this upward pull.

112

SESSION 4

(Bottom of the Pelvis)

BODYREADING

1. Notice the pattern of tension. In the case of knock-knees the tension is on the outside of the lower leg (peroneals), but shifts to the inside in the upper leg (adductors). In bowlegs the tension starts on the inside (tibialis posterior), but shifts to the outside of the upper leg (abductors).

2. When the adductors are overactive, this is often a part of a deep armored contraction running the length of the torso and is evident in the pelvis, diaphragm, and throat. At the pelvis the ischia are usually pulled together. Notice the connection this inward tension on the ischia has with the attachments of the psoas and pelvic floor.

3. When the abductors are overactive -- although the bottom, inner part of the pelvis (ischia) may be open -- the tension usually moves higher into the diaphragm as a part of a continuing outside-inside pattern of tension.

4. When the tension is on the outside in the upper leg, notice that this is often connected with locked knees and that the rectus femorus and vastus lateralis may be stuck together. The rectus serves as a pulley, bringing the top of the pelvis down and contributing to lordosis. We need to lengthen the rectus so that the pelvis can settle back into an upright position.

5. Encourage your client to bend the knees, to feel weak in the knees, to even collapse into the knees. Explore the fears involved in this letting go.

6. Often there is a pattern of one hip being higher, possibly more contracted around the quadratus lumborum with excessive abduction. The other side may then be more open at quadratus lumborum and abductors, but more contracted around the adductors. Explore this possibility by having your model exaggerate the position. Often you will also discover a twist in the torso, toward the more contracted quadratus lumborum.

BODY AREA

Our general aim is to loosen the medial and anterior thigh, giving freedom to the bottom of the pelvis. This will allow sexual feelings moving upward and supply energy to the heart area, throat, mouth and eyes. This release is a condition of connections we will make later from the bottom to the top of the bodymind core.

1. **Lower Leg.** See circled numbers 1 through 4 on illustrations. The working position is on the side, with the higher leg supported by a cushion. As a preparation for working deep on the adductors, it is important to first release the lower leg. In the case of a high arch, the inverters need to lengthen, but when the feet are flat, it will be important to also work on the outside of the lower leg (peroneals). (Much of the needed work on the outside can also be done during the sixth session, while working up the back of the leg). The work on the lower leg is now much deeper than in the second session, and is much selective. You may envelopes which affect the upper leg. And higher, along the leg, if you can find a single effective entrance deep into the medial tibialis posterior, you can release tension which runs all the way through the medial knee to the ischium.

2. **Insertions of medial thigh.** See circled number 5. Just below the medial knee line, many tendons of the upper medial thigh muscles come together in a cluster.

They are surrounded by a bursa sack (gracilis, sartorius, semitendinosis, semimembranosis). Work across and in between these tendons, since their functions tend to be undifferentiated and confused by being stuck together. You can hook the fingers or knuckles of one hand under some tendons, while working with the other hand across the top of the same tendons.

3.   Sartorius. See circled number 7. The position is still with the client on the side. Notice that the sartorius (Taylor's muscle) may be either too far forward toward the rectus femoris (especially in a leg rotated laterally) or too far backward toward the gracilis (when the knees are turned in). You can work along the gracilis, hooking around the sartorius and pulling it in the opposite direction to its misplacement. Have your client flex and laterally rotate the lower leg, during your interaction.

4. Medial Quadriceps. See circled number 6. From this position (side position with upper leg extended posterior at the hip) you can also begin to work with the medial quadriceps, i.e., vastus medialis, vastus intermedius and medial part of the rectus. At the attachments (medial knee) the tissue is shallow, and you will have to work cautiously, but higher along these muscles you can use your elbow or penetrate deep with your fingertips. The interaction is extension of the knee.

5.   Posterior Adductors. See circled number 8. Save the deep middle adductors (pectineus, adductor longus and brevis) until last. First work on the gracilis and muscles posterior to it. Keep your model on the same side but move the upper leg forward, so that it is in a flexed position. You can now work (on the lower leg) from behind your model. First separate the gracilis from the adductor magnus at several points along these muscles. Here you can probably work deep without eliciting much pain. Use your elbow, if your fingers aren't strong enough. The interaction is adduction. (Ask your client to imagine riding a horse and squeezing with the legs).

6.   Separating Flexors and Adductors. Still circled number 8. Separate the adductor magnus from the semimembranosis. Interaction is a combination of adduction and flexion of the lower leg. You can also separate the semitendinosis and semimembranosis, though this work can be handled in the 6th session.

7.   Origins of Flexors and Posterior Adductors. See circled number 8a. The muscles worked with in the preceding numbers 5 and 6 can be released at their origins as well. Bunching the fingers together, work along the ischium asking for either flexion of the lower leg or adduction.

8.   Anterior Adductors. See circled number 9. Now change the position: the same side but the upper leg is again moved backward (extended). Work on the lower leg. You can take a position in front of the model. Imagine the three adductors forming a triangle with the adductor longus the most superficial and at the apex. Begin here between the gracilis and sartorius, weaving with your fingertips until you reach the adductor longus. Proceed toward the base of the triangle and work on the adductors. At the adductor brevis, you can go even deeper. Finally at the base, try going all the way to the attachment of the pectineus. The interaction for all of these is, naturally, adduction.

9.   Attachment of Gracilis. See circled number 10. Now work with the attachment of the gracilis by reaching with both hands under and around it. First going straight down for enough depth, then hooking under and around the gracilis to its attachments on the pubis. Keep your client on the side, if he or she is on the back, the gracilis will be too stretched. The interaction is adduction.

114

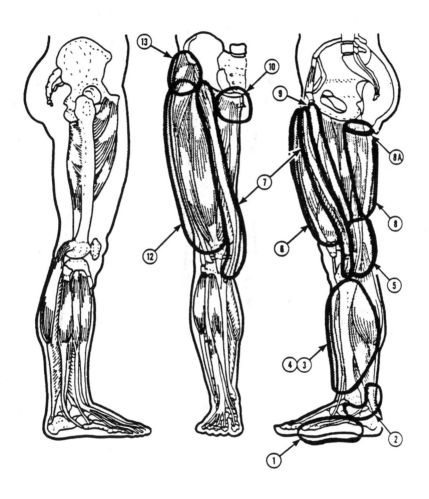

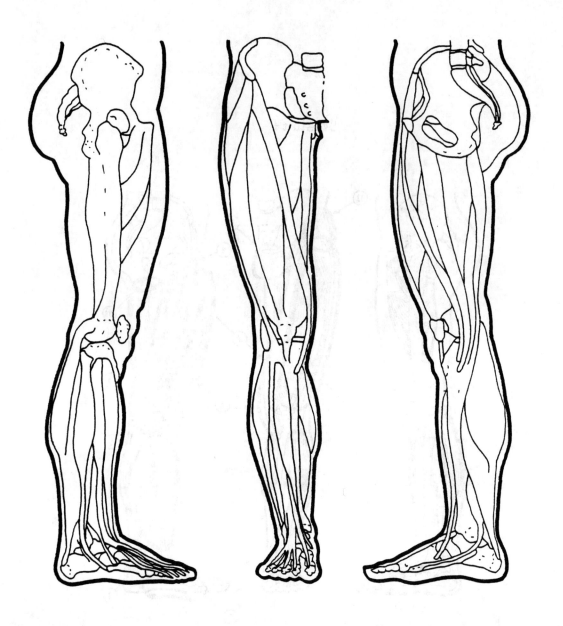

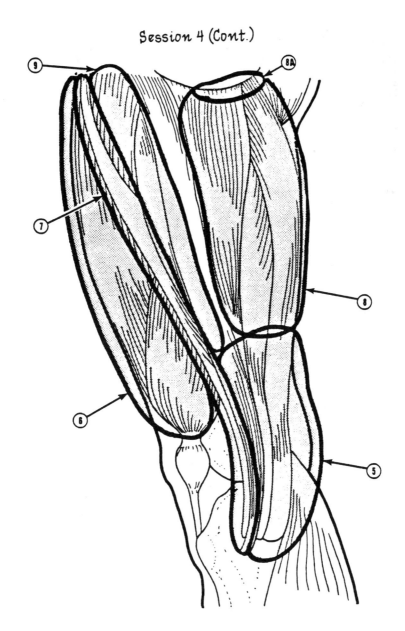

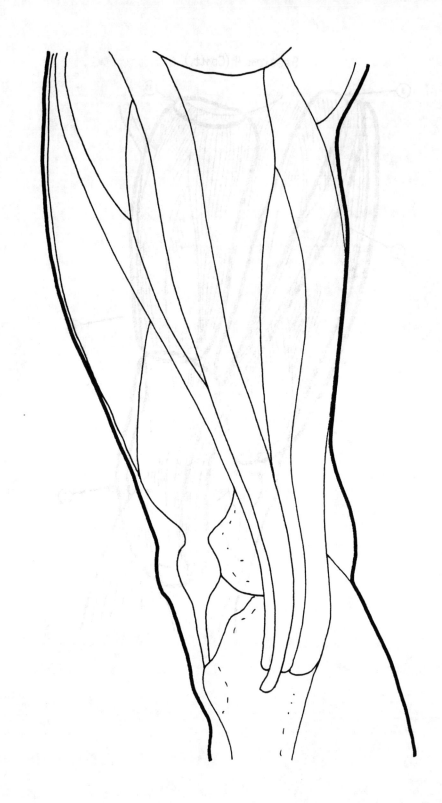

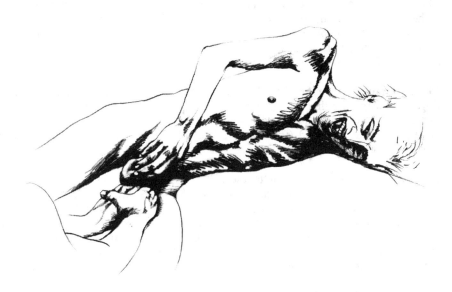

Even when working with an extrinsic (surface) muscle such as the gracilis, the practitioner encourages movement of the pelvis from inside by gentle contraction and relaxation of the psoas, which lies deep in the pelvic bowl and functions as an intrinsic muscle. This often prompts sexual energy to undulate through the entire body.

BODY READING

Up to this point the work has been on the medial lower leg and thigh. Have your client stand so that you can see what's happening. The inner thigh should be fuller; the line from the knee to the pubis, less wavy. Some weight may have shifted to the outside of the thigh, on which you have just worked, and to the inside of the other thigh. The medial arch of the worked leg may also be supporting more weight.

10. Anterior and Lateral Quadriceps. See circled number 12. Now you are ready to work with the other parts of the quadriceps (rectus femoris and vastus lateralis). With the client lying on the back, work across the attachment of the rectus (especially in the case of locked knees). If the rectus is relatively free, proceed to the lateral thigh and separate the rectus and vastus lateralis. Here you can use either the flat of your elbow (not at knee, since that would prevent interacting movement of the knee, but higher along the thigh), or your fingertips or knuckles, perhaps with the knees slightly bent, and supported by a small pillow. Interaction is extension at the knee. Continue along lateral thigh. If you move a little further to the outside, you can also help free the vastus from the iliotibial tract.

11. Anterior Superior Thigh. See circled number 13. At the top work with fingertips deep on either side of the rectus. Here you will be separating the rectus and sartorius, on one side, and the rectus and vastus or vastus and tensor fascia lata, on the other side. You will need (from your client) plenty of flexion and rotation at the hip to get at this complex of envelopes.

12. Origin of Rectus. Go on to the superior process of the iliac spine. There you can work with the origin of the rectus. All this work around the rectus is extremely important in giving the pelvis a chance to lengthen in front, and thus in flattening a sway back. Of course, in the case of lordosis there is a shortening of the back as well, but the job of lengthening and broadening the lower back in the 6th session cannot be effective, unless there is sufficient lengthening of the rectus (on the front of the pelvis) in the fourth session.

HALF WAY READING

Be sure to look at your client after finishing one half. Look for more weight on the medial arch. Also look for an even rounding out of the whole thigh. Also the knee is often more flexible, but since the work is focused on one part of the leg, the knee, in bending more, may turn somewhat inward or outward. A balancing out of the forces acting on the knee will come as the work progresses in other sessions.

OTHER HALF

Follow the same procedure on the other leg. Although this is the more difficult (tighter, more disorganized) leg, it should be more ready to open, especially if you have encouraged the release of feelings during work of the first leg.

NECK AND BACK: As in other sessions.

FINAL FINE ENERGY

During the finishing cycles of charging and discharging breathing, make sure that the energy is not stuck along the channel from the bottom of the pelvis to the throat. Work toward an awareness of this connection of the pelvis with the throat. Images can help: threads or strings that pull gently from bottom to top; a tube of colored energy from the genitals and anus to the throat, etc. Acceptance of the basal chakra in balance with the other body energies is the key, whether this be giving more importance to a neglected pelvis, or less importance to an overactive pelvis. Suggest that with one hand your client hold the genitals, and with the other suck the thumb.

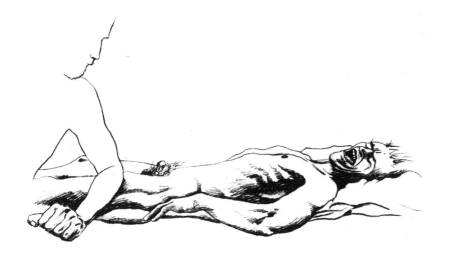

SESSION 5

(Upper Anterior Pelvis)

BODY READING

1. When the pelvis is tilted forward (lordosis), the genitals are often hidden and protected and may store an excess of energy. Work toward the opening and expression of this energy, the acceptance of this sexual power. The extrinsic muscles need to be softened. The intrinsic muscles (e.g., psoas, obturator internus) need to be strengthened.

2. When the pelvis (top) is tilted backward, there is often a lack of energy. There can be an overthrusting forward of the genitals, and at the same time, a closing down in the anus. Work with the quieting of the sexual energy and the release of anal anger. In this case you may also find a great deal of tension in the hamstrings where they pull down on the posterior pelvis.

3. Notice (as in session 4) that a twisted pelvis involves an unevenness of strength between the right and left psoas, which in turn, may have a spinning effect on the spine, or may be involved with tension in the adductors on one side. Sometime a stringy psoas (in spasm without the capacity to function appropriately) will exert a downward pull (forward tilt at top) on one side of the pelvis, while the iliacus on the other side may contract upward, with the help of the obliques and quadratus lumborum.

4. Notice the relation between the tilt of the pelvis and tension in the abdominus rectus and thorax. When the top of the pelvis is tilted forward the chest may be high and overinflated, and the belly dumped forward, though often the abdominal wall will overcompensate in an attempt to pull the contents back inside the pelvic bowl. Often, when the top of the pelvis is tilted backward, the chest is collapsed and the abdomen flat and hard.

BODY AREAS

The main goal is to release and activate the iliopsoas. In order to make the iliopsoas available for this work, one must open and lift the chest, and lengthen the abdominal muscles.

1. Attachments of Abdominus Rectus on the Ribs. See circled number 1. Begin with the client on the back. Make sure there is enough charge or discharge and an adequate connection between diaphragmatic and upper chest breathing before begin ning to work directly on these attachments. Whether done with knuckles or fingers, these strokes have to be deep and slow enough to go between and over the ribs. Working diagonally across the muscle upward toward the mid line, lengthens one half of the rectus at a time.

WORK SYMMETRICALLY

Use one or two strokes on one side, then on the other. This is the case for all the strokes of this session.

2. Attachments of Pectoralis Major. See circle 3. After working both sides of the rectus, continue working diagonally, but now across the fibers of the pectoralis where it attaches along the breast bone. This helps complete the lengthening of the abdominus rectus by encouraging the chest to lift.

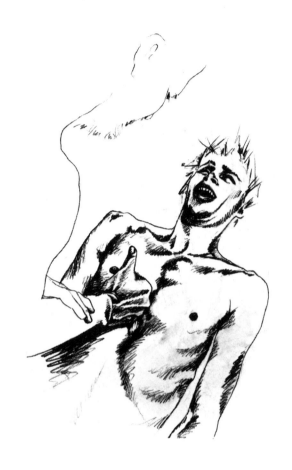

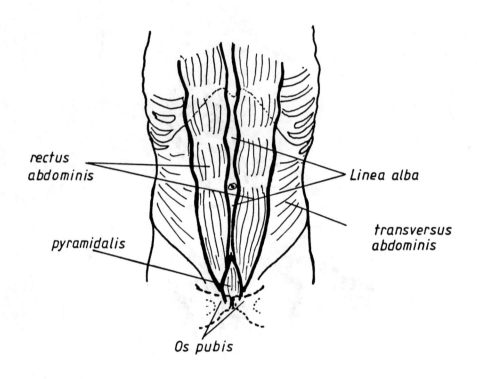

rectus
abdominis

Linea alba

transversus
abdominis

pyramidalis

Os pubis

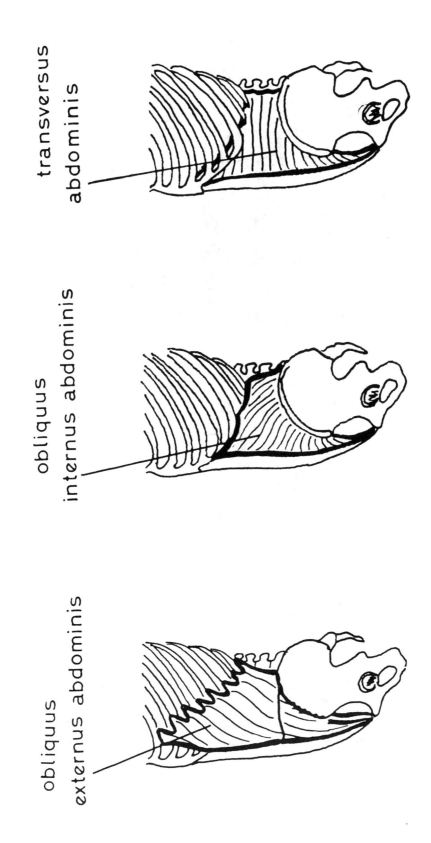

obliquus
externus abdominis

obliquus
internus abdominis

transversus
abdominis

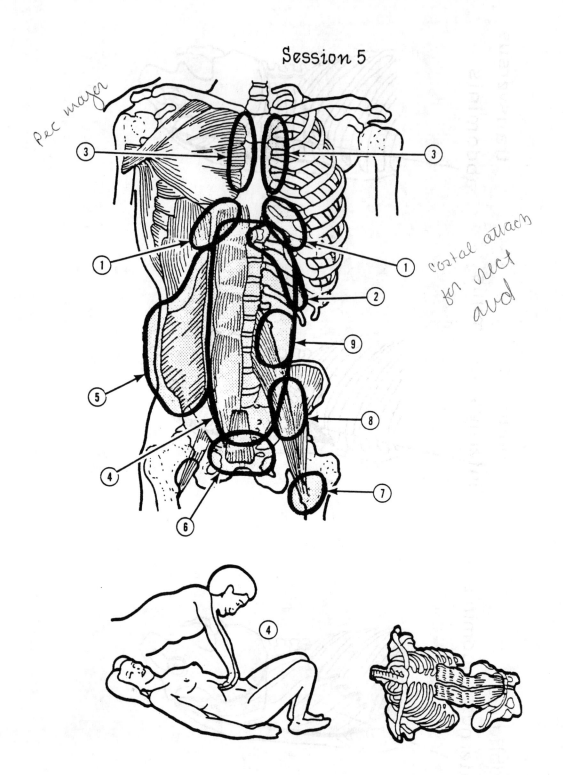

Pec mayer

costal attach
for rect
abd

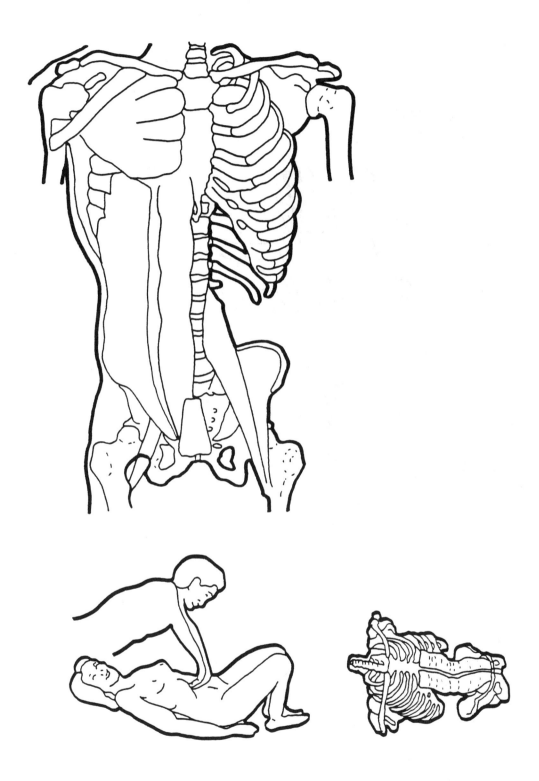

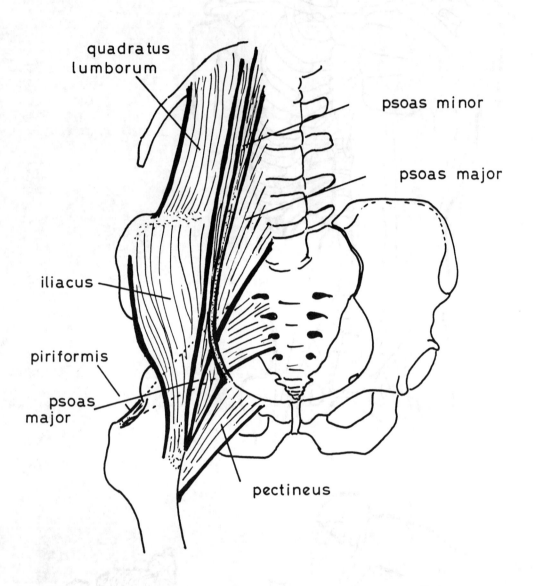

quadratus lumborum

psoas minor

psoas major

iliacus

piriformis

psoas major

pectineus

3. **Pectoralis Minor.** In some cases you may wish to rework (after the work of session 3) the origin and insertions of the pectoralis minor. In cases where the chest is collapsed and the shoulders are rounded, work not only around the coracoid process, but also go to the insertions along the ribs. You need to be deep and exact; twist your knuckles or fingers slightly at the insertion. The shoulder is moved forward.

4. **Diaphragmatic Area.** See circle 2. Expansion of the entire thorax is needed (along with lengthening of the rectus abdominus) in order to give enough space to activate the psoas. Reach under the floating ribs, while supporting their lateral side with your other hand. With your fingertips reach upward and hook inward toward the attachments of the diaphragm. Continue with similar strokes progressing toward the linia alba. The attachments of the diaphragm will be more available as you approach the sternum. If the model curls the pelvis up without contracting the belly and exhales (or pants shallow and high in the chest), your hand can more easily go under the ribs toward the diaphragm. Do the other side. If the belly is too hard, try softening the obliques and abdominus (the next two body areas), before entering the diaphragm.

5. **Obliques.** See circle 5. When there is a tendency toward excessive discharge (collapsing and weak in the front), not only the abdominus, but also the obliques will be tight and short. (It may seem paradoxical that in weakness there will be such a hard contraction, but these muscles are using up a lot of energy that isn't available to the whole person). Cross your hands, back to back, using the fingertips in opposite directions to stretch the tissue toward and away from the floating ribs. This back handed leverage will transfer the force to your fingertips, and spare the floating ribs and the ilium unnecessary pressure. You may need several of these strokes on both sides to open very blocked, lateral and posterior, diaphragmatic breathing.

6. **Pubic Attachment of Abdominus (and pyramidalis).** See circle 6. Before working directly with the abdominus, we loosen both ends of the rectus. We have already worked with the attachments above. We can now directly work on the pubic bone. Straddle the pelvis in a standing position. Bend in the knees, using your weight to press the fingers against the superior border of the pubic bone. As your model rocks the pelvis gently, press from side to side along the bone. Do not exert pressure against the bladder, rather work against the superior surface of the pubis, where the rectus attaches. If the model tightens the abdominus, you won't be able to do these strokes.

7. **Abdominus Rectus.** See circle 4. Straddle your model, facing the feet. Bend in the knees, hooking the abdominus above the pubic hair line. After hooking (the abdominus is relatively flat), pull your fingers diagonally in large zigzags across both halves of the abdominus. You will need many such strokes to cover the entire abdominus up to the thorax. It may help to have your client curl the pelvis (without using the abdominus) as you pull upward.

8. **Separate Abdominus from Transversus (scoop-di-doo).** In giving more space to the belly, it's important to unglue the abdominus from the transversus. This will allow the transversus to balloon all the way around the body during diaphragmatic breathing. Drop the elbows low enough, so that you can scoop up the abdominus with your knuckles.
(Your head will have to go down to your model's belly if you are to get enough power under your wrists).

9. **Insertion of the Iliopsoas.** See circle 7. Consider the pull exerted through the iliopsoas. If one side is more pulled down and the area is more closed around the lesser

trochanter (e.g. there is more adduction), start with the other side, which is more open. Use the side saddle position. With fingers bunched together, find the area between the gracilis and sartorius, just above the insertion of the pectineus, which allows you to penetrate directly medially toward the femor. After you have gone deeper, turn slightly upward until you can feel the lesser trochanter, then press against the attachment. A rocking movement of the pelvis will help you feel movement of the tendons of the iliopsoas. The femoral nerve is in this area. Go slowly at first, but at a certain point simply do it, while encouraging your model to express the pain. Due to the sensitivity of the area, you may not be able to reenter during this session.

10. Body of the Psoas. See circle 8. Now to wake up the psoas. We have created space around the psoas and have loosened its insertions. By directly strumming its body we can not only relax its chronic spastic condition, we can also give it a new responsiveness. With the client on the back and the opposite knee bent for support, practice a movement in which the client moves the ankle and knee, drawing the knee up to a bent position along side the other knee. When the knee is fully bent, the pelvis is rolled up, keeping the belly loose, then rolled back, and the leg is lowered (knee straightened) to the original position. Your stroke begins with the beginning of this pelvic movement; your fingers pressing across the psoas (be sure you are above the ovaries) with maximum pressure being exerted when the pelvis is rolled up. You will be interacting with the contraction and stretching of the psoas. Try different angles, to make sure you have made good contact. If there is a sharp pain as your fingers enter the abdomen, release your pressure and try again. Often there are pockets of gas in the intestines, which will move out of the way. Try the same slightly higher and closer to the ilium and you will contact the iliacus. See circle 9.

11. Lumbar Stretch With Psoas Curl. If the extrinsics are relaxed, the psoas will gently contract, without one having to arch the back. The model's back is flat, the knees are bent. The pelvis is gently curled, using the psoas, while simultaneously, you hook your fingers on either side of the lumbar spine and pull downward. (This means you have to reach under the torso of your model with both hands). The cooperation of the intrinsics and extrinsics allows the back to lengthen and broaden, while having a reciprocal relaxing and strengthening effect on the psoas. The stretch occurs just outside (posterior to) the origins of the psoas along the lumbar spine.

12. Neck and Back. Usual strokes.

FINAL BODY READING

Notice how abdominal and thoracic breathing are more together. The front of the body will be noticeably longer, the chest much higher. If the rectus is still locked (4th session), there may be, during the 5th session, a lengthening of the belly and lifting of the chest, but the lordosis may actually be worse. This means that either the work of the 4th session has to be repeated, then followed by part of the psoas work of session 5; or that more work on the rectus can be incorporated in session 6 and the psoas reworked at the end of session 6.

FINAL FINE ENERGY

Help connect the movement of the chest with the movement of the pelvis and head. After session four it was important to connect the pelvis and throat, without focusing too much on the mid-chest. Now it is important to help your model feel a rocking release in the mid chest with each exhalation. Try out gentle sighing, until the chest and psoas can vibrate together.

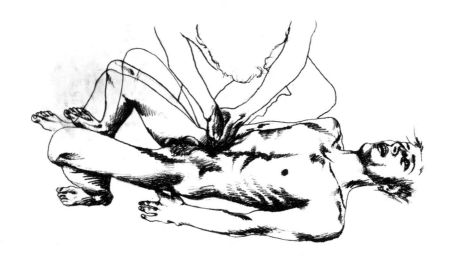

SESSION 6

(Posterior Pelvis)

BODYREADING

1. Notice whether the buttocks are tucked in and the ass tight, or whether the buttocks protrude with the genitals hidden in front. Help your client to exaggerate the position and to get in touch with whatever feeling may be locked in these largely unconscious positions. When the buttocks are tucked, there may be lots of tension in the hamstrings; when the buttocks are high there will be more tension in the lower back and sacrum.

2. When the cheeks are contracted into dimples along the posterior femor, notice the connection with the iliotibial tract and with the lateral gluteals. This tension in the buttocks is also often connected with tension in the sacrum. You may find a little triangular patch of tissue on the sacrum which reflects the tension running through the legs and buttocks, the result of a pattern of tension that shifts from inside to outside and back inside (e.g., inside the knees, outside the buttocks, inside on the sacrum).

3. When the legs are rotated laterally from the hips (not the knees), there will be tension deep in the rotators (piriformis, obturator internus and externus, gemelli, quadratus femoris). This may not always be obvious in the external form of the buttocks, since the tension lies very deep. Even in the case of legs that are relatively straight or medially rotated, there may be considerable compensating, i.e., counter tension in the lateral rotators, especially after you have released a good deal of the tension in the medial rotators.

BODY AREAS

Sessions 4 and 5 generally lengthen the front of the body (e.g. in session 4 the rectus femoris is worked at both origin and insertion and in session 5 the abdominus rectus is lengthened, while the chest is lifted). Since the front and back of the body are in an agonistic-antagonistic relation, prior to session 6 tension will have shifted to the back of the body. Session 6, like other even sessions (excepting 4), will bring more overall balance in the body than odd sessions. After 6 the tension will shift to the neck and head, although the legs and torso will be in a relative balanced release both in front and back.

1. Preparatory Work on the Legs.

   A. Peroneals and Lower Leg. See circles 1 through 4. The release of the deeper myofascial wrappings of the lower leg was begun in session 4, we continue this work, focusing on the lateral and posterior parts of the lower leg. While emphasizing the lateral part of the leg (peroneals, lateral part of soleus and gastrocnemius), you may be able to penetrate both sides of the leg, simultaneously also reworking the medial side. Here the knuckles or fingers slide in between and separate the muscles from both side.

   B. Gastrocnemius. See circle 5. Divide the gastrocnemius, using two hands (knuckles or fingertips in opposite directions), in preparation for going deeper in the region just underneath the popliteal fossa. But let this separating be in a downward direction. The plantar flexors generally need to lengthen downward, not shorten upward.

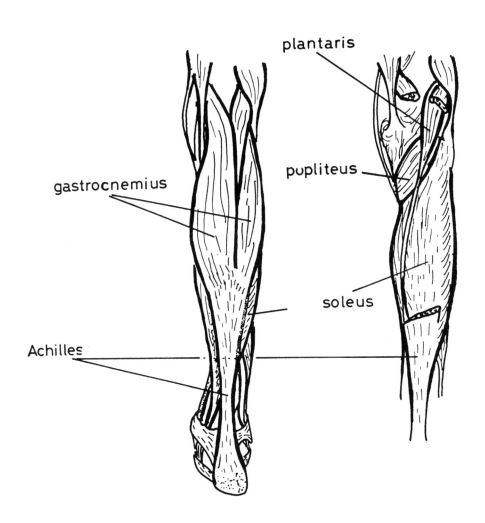

plantaris

gastrocnemius

popliteus

soleus

Achilles

133

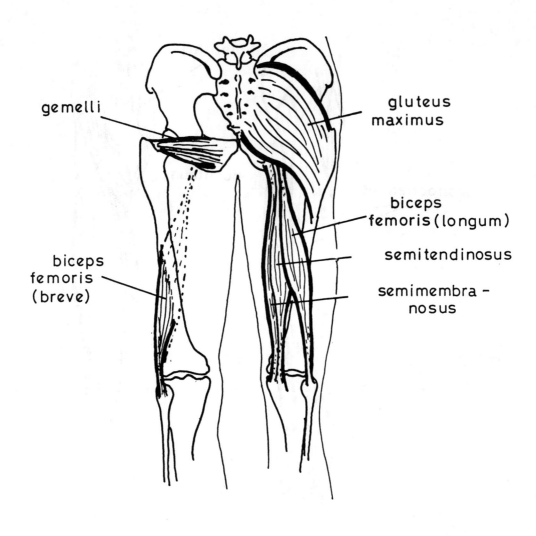

gemelli

gluteus
maximus

biceps
femoris (longum)

semitendinosus

biceps
femoris
(breve)

semimembra -
nosus

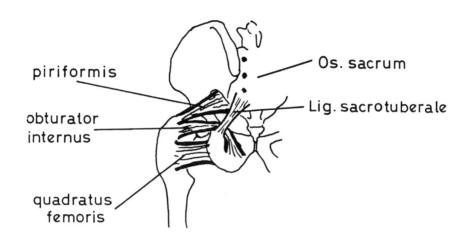

piriformis

obturator
internus

quadratus
femoris

Os. sacrum

Lig. sacrotuberale

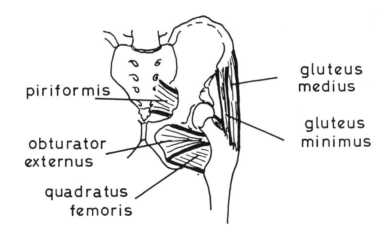

piriformis

obturator
externus

quadratus
femoris

gluteus
medius

gluteus
minimus

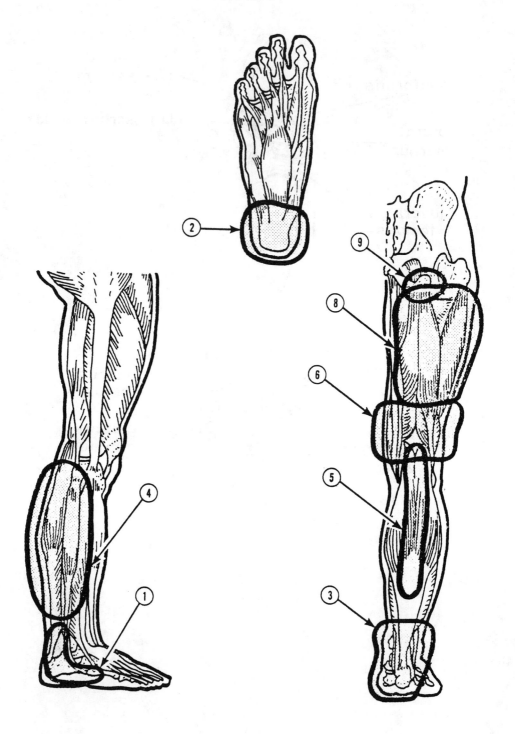

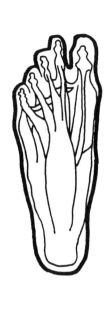

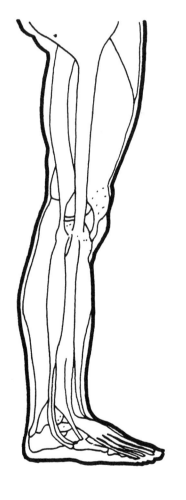

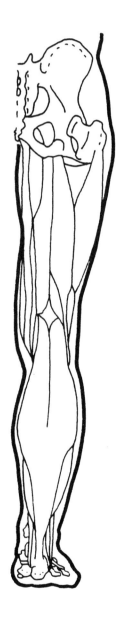

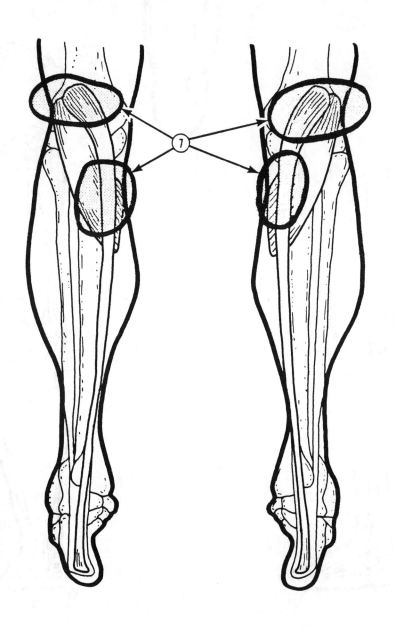

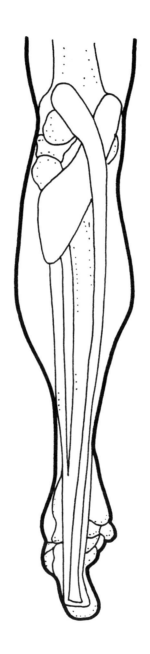

C. Back of the Knee. See circle 7. The plantaris lies one level below the gastrocnemius, and the popliteus lies still a level deeper. You need direct penetrating (but slow) strokes to get sufficient depth. Work on the attachments of both these muscles and at the same time on the posterior lateral part of the knee. This is a bony area that calls for steady, powerful knuckles. Next work on the body of the plantaris with fingertips or two pointed knuckles. The interactive movement is plantar flexion. To reach the insertion of the popliteus, roll the leg slightly medial and use the fingertips to press along the tibia, during medial rotation at the knee.

D. Above the Knee. See circle 6. Avoid the popliteal fossa but hook the fingertips of both hands symmetrically on the medial border of the hamstrings, and continue deep under the hamstrings to the origins of the gastrocnemius. Keep the depth and continue the stroke across the hamstrings (semitendinosis on one side and biceps femoris on the other side). The interactive movement is plantar flexion. This work will clearly open the knee in two directions: upward into the back of the legs and downward to the achilles tendon, (a tremendous overall lengthening of the whole leg).

E. Biceps Femoris. See circle 8 and 9. When the ass is tucked under, the hamstrings will be shortened, pulling toward their origins but also downward toward their insertions. This pattern can be connected with hyperextension of the back (overcontraction of the sacrospinalis) and the inability of the spine to bend forward in graceful, rolling movements. The insertion of the short head of the biceps lies along the lateral part of the leg, a few centimeters above the knee. You can use your elbow in a very short stroke, shifting and twisting slightly, while the interactive movement is straightening and relaxing the knee. (An alternative interaction is to have the knee completely bent and let the heel move back and forth toward the buttocks). You may wish to work on the body of the biceps separating its stringy fibers, or strumming across it in provoking, but lengthening movements. Finally work on its origin at the inferior ischium. The elbow will probably not reach this corner. Bunched fingertips can strum, while the knee straightens.

2. Rotators. See circles 10 through 12. The lateral rotators of the leg are obviously overcontracted when the legs are splayed outward in Donald Duck or Charlie Chaplin fashion. (The feet may be turned out from the knee, however, without the upper leg being laterally rotated). Sometimes, when the leg is relatively straight, there may be lots of mutually compensating tension in both the medial and lateral rotators. In this case be sure to rework the medial rotators after working in the sciatic notch on the lateral rotators.

A. Piriformis. It Lies in the upper part of the sciatic notch. Use the elbow to massage gently the area, gradually going deeper. When applying maximum pressure, explore different angles, since the tension is variable along the length of this muscle. Interaction is rotation of the whole leg from the hip.

B. Obturators, and Gemelli. These muscles originate deep in the pelvis and are intrinsic muscles which have a lot to do with pelvic stability and freedom of the legs to move in parallel lines from the hips. Use the same style elbow stroke with rotation. You may want also to reach the obturator internus by another stroke with the fingers high along the medial border of the ischium.

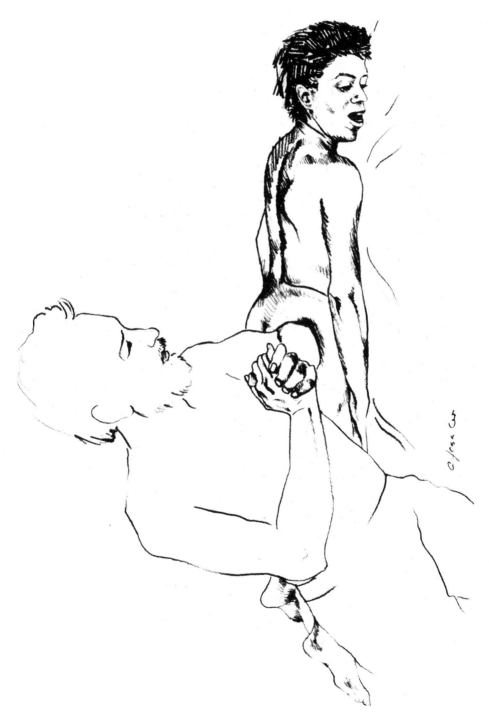

C. Quadratus Femoris. To reach these short muscles between the lateral ischium and medial femur, use the fingertips. You may have to use prying movements -- against the ischium or against the femur or upward toward the sciatic notch -- in order to free these, not readily available, muscles.

HALFWAY BODYREADING

Look at the position of the leg. Has a laterally rotated leg straightened? Also consider the shape of the buttocks. The worked on buttock may now be rounder and fuller. There may also be a visible lengthening of one side of the back.

3. Sacrum. See circle 13 and 14. Connect the sciatic notch and sacrum with strokes pulling downward over the superior edge of the notch into the notch. Next work on the sacrum. Use a great deal of pressure with a flat elbow, pushing downward and toward the mid line, along the major areas of the sacrum. This thickened and hardened tissue can, with time and work, become so soft it will slide off the sacrum to which it has become glued through many years of unawareness and bunched immobility. You may want to bend your model over the table with the belly on the table top and knees on the floor. From this position a slight rocking movement of the pelvis can also help reorganize the tissue of the sacrum.

4. Sacrospinalis. See circle 15. It is important, before working on the coccyx, to loosen the back, at least up to the mid-thoracic hinge, perhaps even as far as the neck. Use downward diagonal strokes. Begin with the elbow flat, and as your pressure reaches the middle of the muscle, sharpen the angle of your elbow such that, finally, you use the point of the elbow next to the spine. Do one side at a time. The tissue around the sacrospinalis tends to be too spread out across the back and holds the ribs too flat. As you work the tissue toward the spine, the sacrospinalis will come more together, becoming rounder and softer. The ribs will then be free to move at the spinal processes, rounding toward the back and front. The whole torso then is fuller and rounder and less square, less flat in front and back.

5. Coccyx. See circle 16. The bones of the body guide the tissue which in turn distributes the weight of the body. The coccyx is a kind of a rudder for the spine and when it is bent upward or sideways, or in rare cases comes too far posterior (is not bent enough), the distribution of weight in the tissues of the pelvis and legs is confused. Also this is a key area for introverted, stubborn feelings, and release and reorganization of the tail can bring a profound, deep seated relaxation and feeling of well being throughout bodymind.

6. Psoas. You may wish to rework the psoas. Often, after the release of the back, the psoas will respond even more completely to deep stimulation. You may want to combine work on the psoas in front with work on muscles in the back, e.g., obturator internus, in order to create a subtle, pelvic balance between front and back.

FINAL BODYREADING

The two most significant changes will be the position of the legs (more parallel) and the softening of the sacrum. The sacrum accumulates stress and tends to cut itself off from the buttocks. There should now be a much more continuous flow of tissue from the hamstrings up through the sacrum. This may be evident in a diaphragmatic breath which ripples through the ribs and buttocks.

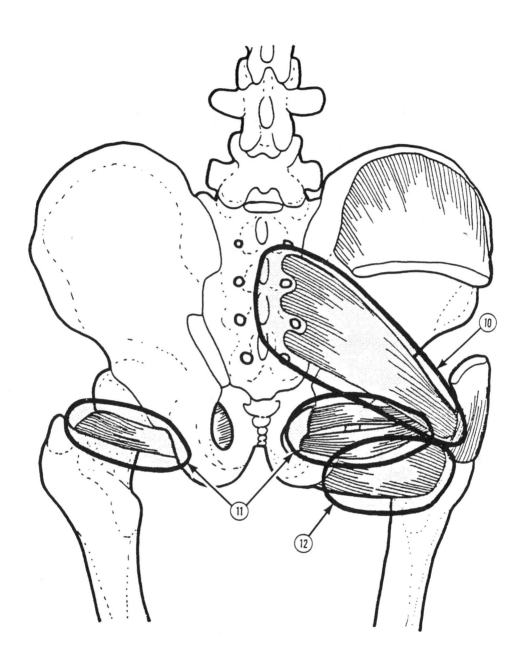

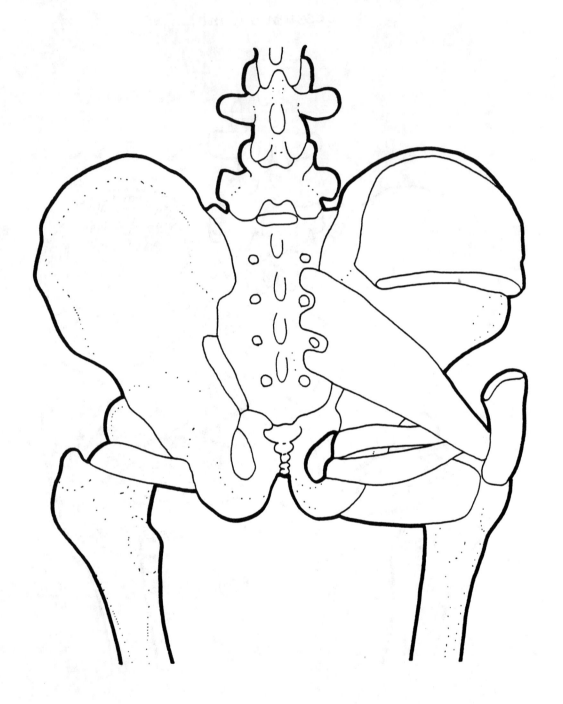

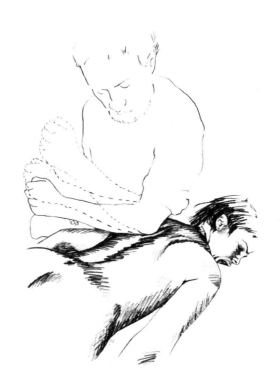

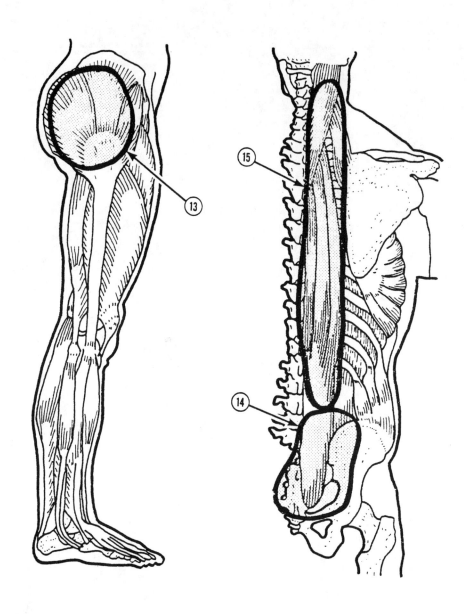

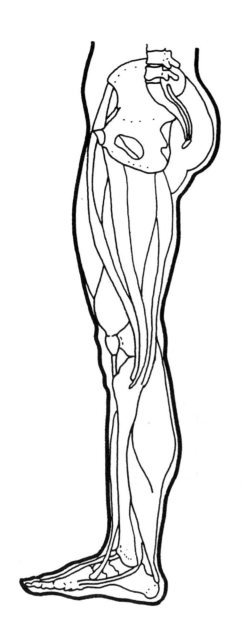

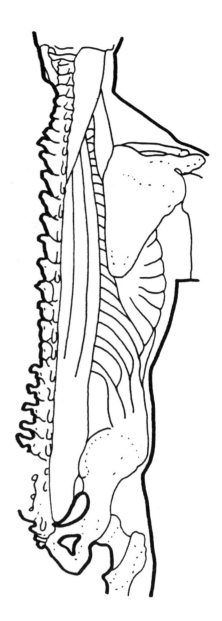

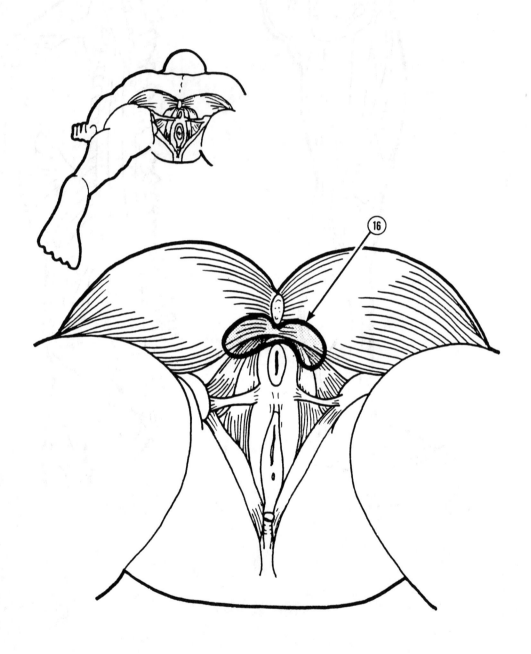

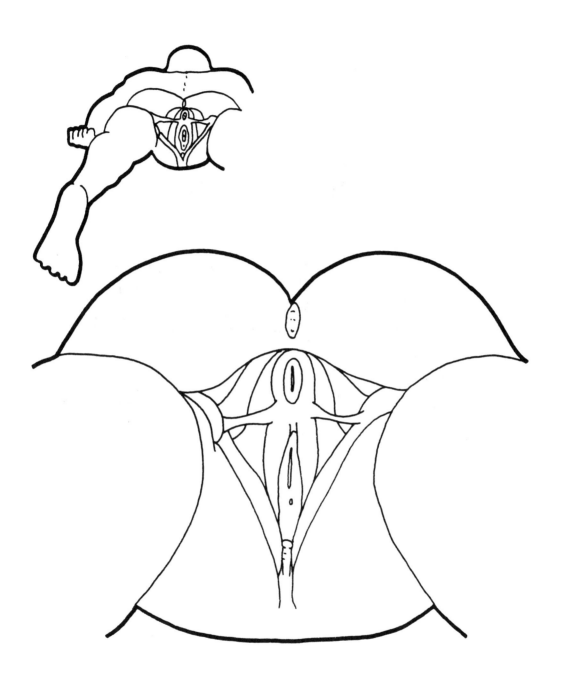

149

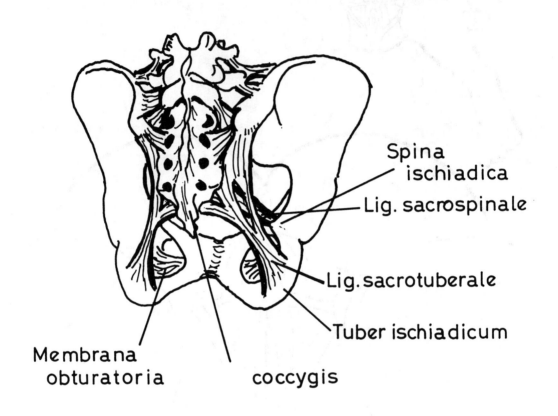

Spina
ischiadica

Lig. sacrospinale

Lig. sacrotuberale

Tuber ischiadicum

Membrana
obturatoria

coccygis

FINAL FINE ENERGY

From the time of the anal stage of development, we separate our deep seated resentments from our conscious attitudes. With the expression of this repressed anger, we have a chance to let power stream through our whole body. Receptivity and assertiveness now are simply different directions for the same feeling, which we can take in or express outward through our extremities and torso. Work toward the recognition that anger is diffuse, expansive, circulating energy rather than merely repressed and contracted resentment. Connect coccyx Gv1 and occiput Gv15. Use both The Doors of Life and Windows to the Sky.

PHASE IV: RELEASE OF THE HEAD AND NECK

(Session 7)

GENERAL PURPOSE

Now we want to free the cervical vertebrae, allowing the neck and head to move into alignment with the pelvis; to free the emotions around the eyes, mouth, and throat so that feelings from other parts of the body can be easily and completely expressed through the head.

BODYTYPE

1.   **Oral types** accumulate either a weakness (mouth open) or overcontraction (clinched jaw). We are looking for a light bite which gives boundaries to what is taken in, but also permits sucking in what is needed. Some oral types may have the chin lifted and thrust forward. Slow everything down, encourage watching what is happening.

2.   **Very Right-Sided individuals** may have an overdeveloped masculine side which controls the feminine side. Active Left- Sided individuals may feel guilt about or conflict with the right side. During the work, encourage a gestalt dialogue between the two sides. Remember that K27 is good for this imbalance.

3.   **Some Rigid types** may have relatively straight cervical vertebrae but be extremely tight and inflexible in the anterior neck muscles. The sternocleidomastoids may be stiff and large, and the masseter clinched. There may be repressed orality, if they were weaned too early. At the right moment encourage them to feel their needs, to suck and bite.

4.   **Schizoid types** have lots of energy in the head, but it is unfocused. Work with the eyes. Use eye contact and eye exercises (eyes follow the movements of a penlight or finger). Don't allow any fantasizing or drifting away; keep them present.

THOUGHT AND AFFIRMATION

The head is too often the center of deliberation, consideration, and reflexion. It is important to accept the head as simply another part of bodymind. Thoughts then do not require effort, struggle, and lots of time; they can be easy, clear and immediate, just like the movement of a leg or arm. Try "I'm thinking with my whole self;" "My ideas are clear and complete;" "I'm certain of what I am now contacting;" "I can sit on my head;" "I can run with my ears."

MANIPULATIONS

1.   **Depth.** The neck holds a maze of muscle, many layers one over the other. This work is very deep, and very slow.

2.   **Precision.** There are many fragile nerves and vessels in the neck and head. Be sure where and how you want to work. The fingers, being the most exact instruments of your body, will do most of the work of this session.

3. If some parts of the neck and head are too highly charged to do all the work in one session, the session can be repeated. Or if certain essential parts can be released
(gums, tongue, cervical vertebrae) the postponed parts can be incorporated in sessions 8, 9, and 10.

MOVEMENT AWARENESS

Many people do not have consciousness of how the head can turn on its vertical axis. Use the Feldenkrais exercise in which the model looks with the eyes only at one shoulder tip but turns the head the opposite direction. This exercise can help with getting more distance between the ears and shoulders. Work with the image of a milkmaid's collar, holding two buckets on either side. This helps give a sense of the shoulders having a flat top, and being anchored. Also work with the idea that the chin can fall a little, while the back of the neck elongates. A lifting string attaches at the back of the head, not near the front which would lift the chin. As the chin falls and the back of the neck lengthens, the chest lifts with an inhalation. Compare the needy types who collapse the chest and lift the chin in search of the unobtainable.

MERIDIANS AND POINTS

Brushing the upper yang meridians will bring a lot of energy to the neck and head. The windows to the sky are essential before, during and after this session (Cs1, Cv22, S9, Li18, Si16, Tw16, B10, Gv16, L3). After working an entire session on the head, be sure to reground your model by using S36 and other points on the lower body.

CHAKRAS

Use the higher centers as enhancers of the other centers. Do not think of the third eye or uppermost chakra as an escape from the other chakras, but as their culmination. Use a tone meditation Lam, Vam, Yam, Ham, Ram, Om for ascending and descending through the chakras.

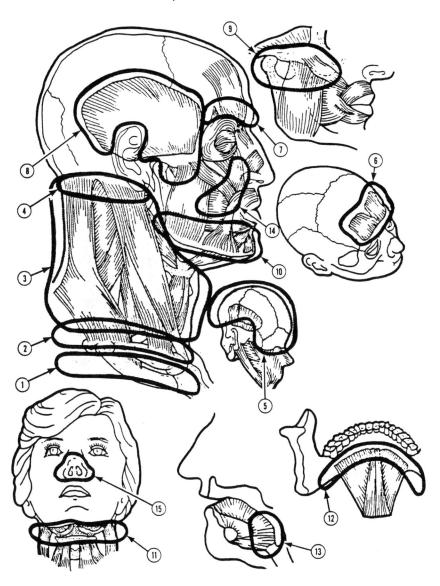

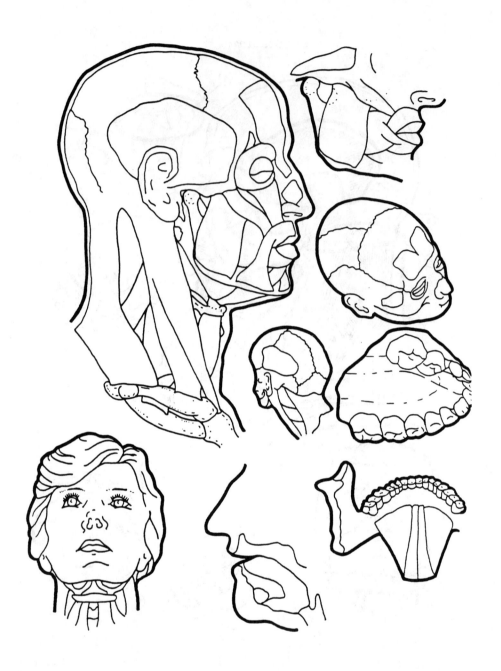

SESSION 7

(Head and Neck)

BODYREADING

1. The forward angle in the cervical vertebrae will usually duplicate the angle in the lumbar vertebrae. This angle cuts off the consciousness between the head, torso, and neck. Most people do not realize that the neck can rest easily on the spine, such that there is connection all the way from the atlas and axis down to the coccyx.

2. Notice that the neck sometimes is advanced by being pulled forward to the clavical, that is, the base of the whole neck is too far forward. In this case the trapezius may be wrapped like a cobra hood over the shoulders, and there may be the beginning of a dowager's hump at the 7th cervical. Lots of work on the upper chest and clavicle will be needed. In other cases, the neck may be pulled more forward at the mid-cervical vertebrae or the chin jutted forward. In these cases more work is needed inside the mouth and with the capitis muscles, which will be short in the back of the neck.

BODY AREAS

1. Subclavicular Area. See circle 1. Preliminary reworking of the pectoralis major and minor may be necessary, before working under the clavicle. The muscles of the neck are enclosed in fascia that extends under the clavicle and is connected with the first rib. Slide your fingers against the third and second ribs and move your pressure upward under the clavicle toward the first rib. The client can turn the neck and tilt it from side to side.

2. Supraclavicular Area. See circle 2. One side at a time: Using the broad part of the thumbs (one of the rare occasion that the thumbs are better than other parts of the hand), pull across the two tendons of the sternocleidomastoid, while your client turns the head. Continue with the thumb along the omohyoid, scalenus anterior, and medialis, etc. all the way out to the shoulder tip. As you get further toward the shoulder, you can exert more pressure into the anterior trapezius.

3. Anterior and Lateral Neck. See circles 3 and 4.

A. Begin with the usual neck strokes (usually at the end of each session) transverse to the muscles of the neck.

B. Work now to separate the longitudinal muscles of the neck. Using the fingers or knuckles, work along the muscles from the clavicle to their attachments on the head -- sternocleidomastoid, omohyoid, scaleni. These strokes are not transverse but along and in between the muscles, in order to get good separation in their functions. When you work with the sternocleidomastoid, be careful, on the medial side, not to press too deeply into the trachea. Also higher at the attachment of the sterno on the mastoid, be careful, on the medial side, to work slowly along the parotid glands. You can work through glands, but much more slowly than through other connective tissue. Have your client turn the neck as you progress to muscles further along the lateral neck.

C. You may need to work thoroughly across the attachments of all these muscles at the mastoid and occiput.

4. Scalp Aponeurosis. See circle 5. The scalp coordinates muscles on the posterior, lateral, and anterior skull, and you need to loosen all of it before working with the temporalis, frontalis and other muscles of the jaw and face. Beginning at the occiput, grip the scalp with an open hand, so that the force is equally distributed between the fingers and the thumb (like playing a whole octave on the piano). While maintaining this grip, shift the whole hand a short distance. Do not pull the fingers along the scalp; move the whole scalp, otherwise you will pull the hair. You can do this with both hands simultaneously. An alternative grip is with all the knuckles and thumb. Cover the scalp in two halves, all the way from the occiput to the frontalis and temporalis, but do not yet do these latter two areas. Help your client get in touch with how the whole scalp can move; how it is connected with muscles all around the head.

5. Frontalis. See circle 6. With the fingertips (both hands) pull over the supraorbital ridge, upward toward the hairline, along the frontalis. Before beginning, have the model practice pullingthe frontalis down by frowning in equal steps to the count of ten. This same muscle movement is used during your pull upward to give a counter-pull in the opposite direction. Instead of the fingers, you can also use the flat of the knuckles to pull up. Show your client how to move the frontalis with the scalp by moving the ears. This helps relieve chronic tension in the forehead and open the bunched worry and concern between the eyebrows. If there are deep vertical worry lines, try a stroke with both knuckles across the forehead, while the client counter-pulls with an inward frown.

6. Temporalis. See circle 8. Notice the fanlike origins of the temporalis around the ear and temples. There may be a lot of anger here, along the gall bladder meridian. Since the skull is thin, and delicate vessels run through these areas, work shallow and slow, beginning at the periphery of the muscle and working toward the insertion. The fingertips of both hands can be used in pushing strokes; or the flat part of the thumbs, if the pressure is not too concentrated. Use zigzagging movements, so that you are sure to pick up the envelope of the temporalis. The client opens and closes the jaw, or grits the teeth slightly.

7. Muscles of the Jaw and Temperomandibular Joint. See circle 9. There is usually a concentration of anger in this area. Before beginning these strokes, you might encourage some growling and biting, to make sure the client is primed to let go of deeper anger, which may begin to come to the surface during the strokes.

>   **A. Origin of Masseter.** The masseter is more superficial than the temporalis, which passes under the zygomatic arch and attaches on the upper process of the mandible. The insertion of the masseter is available just against the zygomatic. Use the thumbs on the forehead for support (standing above the head of the model) and press the fingers upward against the bone, while the client moves the jaw open and closed.

>   **B. Insertion of the Temporalis.** Use the same position and almost the same grip with the fingers. But now drive the fingers deeper and let the pressure be, not against the cheek, but against the mandible. Use the same jaw movement.

>   **C. Body of the Masseter.** You can work directly on the masseter by inserting your first finger (with the pad lateral) between the outside of the teeth and the masseter. Push your finger as far as you can to the back of the teeth. As your client slowly grits the teeth, your finger will be pushed out against the masseter. In this way the model

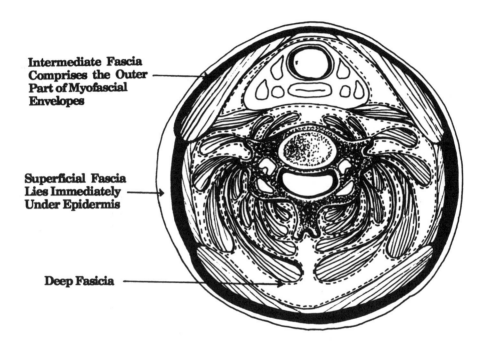

**Intermediate Fascia
Comprises the Outer
Part of Myofascial
Envelopes**

**Superficial Fascia
Lies Immediately
Under Epidermis**

Deep Fasicia

This cross-section of the neck shows an outer superficial layer, an intermediate layer, and deep layer of fascia. The deep fascia is a complicated maze of myofascial sheaths (dashed lines), holding deep and intense emotions. Since the head and neck are an outlet for energy released in other parts of the body, it is important that the practitioner work frequently with these deep, intrinsic structures in the neck.

can regulate the pressure. A good affirmation at this point is "I create and accept my own anger."

D. Insertion of the Masseter. Finally, work directly against the lower mandible with the finger or thumbs. Working with both hands at the same time helps equalize the pressure. You can normally feel a large lump of developed muscle here. It needs lots of work, especially in people who hold back resentment.

8. The Tongue and Cervical Vertebrae. Large groups of muscles in the neck, head, and jaw have been released as a preparation for the most important area of this session. We want to loosen the attachments of the tongue, and then push the tongue posterior, in order to loosen the mid-cervical vertebrae. See circles 11 through 13.

A. The Attachments of the Tongue From Outside. See circle 11. With your position still above the head of the client and somewhat to the side, reach the fingers under the mandible, using the thumb on the lateral edge of the jaw for support, press the fingers against the inner (medial) surface of the jaw and have your model extend and retract the tongue. Be especially slow here, since you will also be sliding through the submaxillary glands. Continue this work on both sides of the jaw and in front, under the chin.

B. The Attachments of the Tongue From Inside. Examine the inside of the mouth. Notice that the formation of the teeth is probably not symmetric. The line of one side may be more narrow than the other. Also the teeth may be too narrow in front or in the back. Usually the shape of the teeth reflects the shape of the pelvis. The tongue attaches along the mandible in the soft gums below the teeth. Reach with your first finger, bracing the hand with the thumb against the outside of the teeth. Move the tissue in short strokes (the pad of the finger tip) toward back of the mouth. This is the direction the tissue needs to release in order to free the back of the neck. Work both sides of the gums all the way back past the last molars. Don't forget the front gums. The goal is to loosen the base of the tongue all along the floor of the mouth. This is usually painful. Give space for the expression of some of the most primal feelings.

C. Shifting of Tongue Posterior. The base of the tongue is connected to deep layers of tissue which wrap around the throat, and envelop the mid-cervical vertebrae. After loosening the attachments of the tongue, this whole complex can be shifted with the tongue toward the vertebrae. Position the head so that the back of the neck is flat and the chin is tucked in. One hand under the occiput will help maintain this position. With the other hand use the first two fingers to flatten the tongue against the floor of the mouth. While clamping down against the floor (don't allow the tongue to bunch toward the back of the mouth), move the tongue backward and somewhat down into the throat. You will be pushing against a gag reflex, so your pressure needs to be secure. Before doing this explain that the breath will be cut off for a few seconds and that there may be the sensation of gagging, but that the whole thing is very brief. Check the back of the neck before and after this work to see if it is freer and fuller.

9. Breadth of Cheeks. See circle 14. In order to be in balance with the mouth, jaw, nose and eyes, the cheeks should be wide. The zygomatic bones can actually move further apart. With the pads of both thumbs, push up and out against the cheeks. Do not drag

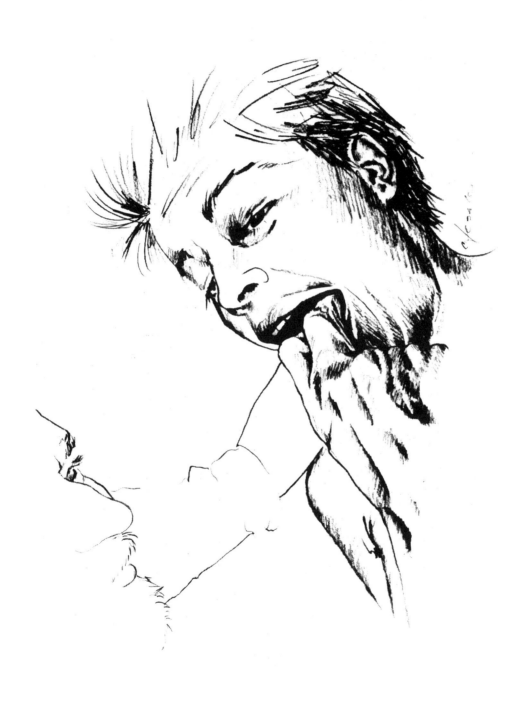

superficial tissue; be securely against the bone. Go slowly; this can be painful. We will discover in advanced PI that the mobility of the zygomatic is important for movement of the sphenoid and freedom of the eyes.

10. Opening the Conchi of the Nose. Inside the nose, on either side , there are three passages, formed by cartiliginous "conchi" (Greek for "scrolls") -- a lower, middle, and upper passage. The septum separates identical structures on both sides. But often one side is more closed than the other, the conchi and septum being broken from accidents or malformed since birth. The walls of the passages may actually be collapsed or stuck together. With slow, accurate pressure, and the release of blocked emotions and thoughts, these passages can be reopened. The balance between the two sides in breathing is important for the heart, (according to both western rhinologists and eastern yogis). Examine the structure of the nose. Sometimes the septum is deviated only at the tip of the nose; sometimes its deviation begins much higher. One side of the nose can be more collapsed or smaller. Also ask whether it is easier to breathe on one side than the other. Start your work on the side more open. Have your model wet your little finger with the mouth. Position yourself on the same side of the body as the side of the nose you are going to enter. Turn the pad of the little finger lateral away from the septum in order to be able to push out on stuck conchae. (If you want to work directly on the septum, reach across and enter the other nostril and push the pad of the little finger medial against the septum). Enter the lower conchae first. Wait for the nostril to open. Suggest to your client images of opening and relaxing around your finger. Gradually advance to the second and third passage. This may require a lot of waiting. Also if the sneeze reflex is activated, do not remove your finger. You will be able to advance slightly, with the relaxation immediately following each sneeze. This work with the nose will open the eyes and make it easier to cry. Also you may reactivate memories associated with the olfactory nerve. Your client may "smell" earlier events. Work with the attendant emotions and attitudes.

NECK

Rework the neck as in other sessions, but now you can go deeper and shift more of the tissue of the neck posterior. Also work with your client in a semi-headstand, moving across the attachments of the capitis muscle at the occiput. This is the same stroke used in session 3, but now is deeper.

BACK

Do as in previous sessions, but you may find it easier to move the sacral tissue, now that the neck is freer.

PSOAS

You will also find the psoas more available now that the neck is freer. Use strokes from session 5.

FINAL BODY READING

Examine the position of both the base of the neck and the mid cervical vertebrae. Often the shift backward is amazing, but don't be discouraged if there seems to be little change in position. The neck is stubborn and you may need to work more on the pelvis before the

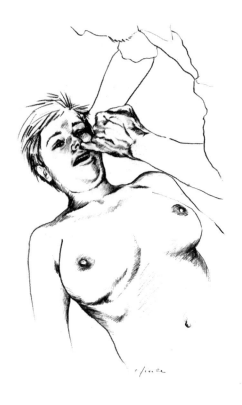

neck is ready to release completely. In any case, you will find the tissue fuller and the neck more mobile.

FINAL FINE ENERGY

1. Focus on the connections between the cervical and lumbar vertebrae. Help your model with images which make the spine one unit from top to bottom. Try the spinal roll exercise (without any manipulations). Show how its possible to lean forward without lifting the chin or arching the back.

2. There is a tendency for the small muscles of the face to lose tone. The pull of gravity, feelings of heaviness and sadness, and chronic overcontraction to the point of weakness cause drooping of the face even in young people. As a kind of fine tuning give your model a few exercises to lift the cheeks or jowls. (These have to be done everyday). These exercises are very precise and need to be studied. See Face Lifting by Exercise, Senta Maria Runge, Allegro Publ Co., P.O. 39892, L.A. 90039

PHASE V: INTEGRATION OF BODYMIND

(Sessions 8, 9, 10)

GENERAL PURPOSE

After the release of armor in individual parts of bodymind -- legs, pelvis, head, etc..-- it is important to focus on bringing these parts together, getting them to function as one unit. The different layers of connective tissue are now free enough to be organized in long planes which flow the entire length of the body. Also the outside layers can be coordinated with the inside layers, such that one layer does not try to compensate for or to protect the other. The focus is also now upon the unity of emotions and thoughts, allowing one feeling or thought to complete itself and to flow into the next. Sessions 8 and 9 divide the bodymind into two halves and 10 works with the whole bodymind structure.

BODYTYPE

Look at the bodymind in terms of symmetric parts: top- bottom, front-back, left-right.

1. Notice whether the structure is more bottom-heavy or top- heavy in deciding with which half to begin. See below decision to be made for session 8. Notice also that a person may be a mixture: partly open on top and partly open on the bottom.

2. Notice the relation of front to back. Many oral and burdened types are contracted in front, while many rigid types are contracted in back.

3. Schizoid types are asymmetric. They do not work in the same way on both sides. Nurture the neglected side.

EMOTION

1. During the release phases of the work, there may have often been very explosive expression of feelings which had long been held back. During the integrative stage, the emotions are just as intense, but there may be less focus on their active expression. The focus is more on being conscious of what is felt, and the balance of one emotion with another.

2. However, in individuals who hold their feelings deep in the core, there may be, in this final stage, still some explosive moments.

3. Focus not only on the acceptance and harmonizing of old emotions, but on the exploration of new feelings. This may caxll for a great deal of support, encouragement and approval.

THOUGHT AND AFFIRMATION

1. As the planes of fascia between the two halves begin to connect, we also begin to open ourselves to more integrated ways of feeling and thinking. I can now say to myself, "I am expansive above, and at the same time, I can support myself below." Or, "I am well grounded, and I can soar." When we integrate ourselves we no longer use one part to manipulate or compensate for another part of ourselves. We begin to realize that we can have both without competition.

2. Gestalt work can be especially beneficial in claiming parts of bodymind. Encourage your client to be active in consciously identifying themselves with the movement and positions of different body parts. They can verbally express themselves from this parts, e.g., "I am now my foot; I'm flat and tired: I refuse to work anymore."

3. In bringing together the above mentioned halves of ourselves, we need to recognize and accept our asymmetry. For example my left side can say to my right side, "It's o.k. that you're more active than me, and don't forget how important I am in smoothing out and softening your actions." Or the top can say to the bottom, "I know that you've always been weaker than me; I'm not going to make lots of demands on you; I'll give you a chance to support me in your own way."

MANIPULATIONS

1. The integration, the organization of overall bodymind, calls for the movement of all three layers of tissue, simultaneously. By using a stroke that is both broad and deep, you can shift more than one layer of tissue at once.

2. Use two handed strokes which organize the tissue in different directions. The direction of movement will depend on what each person needs, but we can illustrate with two general cases. (See "Direction of Movement of Body Segments, Structure A" and "... Structure B").

The most usual structure, A, is one in which there is a pronounced sway in the back. The pelvis in this case needs to lift in the front and drop in the back. (Notice arrows for Structure A). Since the lower back is compensating for the forward tilt of the pelvis, the lower back muscles are contracting downward and our direction of movement is just the opposite, up along the lower back (although down along the sacrum). Higher in the back near the shoulders, however, we want to pull tissue across the trapezius and downward in order to encourage the shoulder girdle to settle back into place (except in cases where the shoulders are already pulled too far back). Notice also that the chin is usually tilted up, being pulled from the back by downward contractions of the capitis muscles. In this case we want to work up the mid-posterior neck up to the occiput.

In Structure B note that our work is up most of the posterior body. The hamstrings are pulling down, the ass is tucked under, the lower back muscles are hyperextending. All along the back our direction of movement is upward against these downward contractions.

In the front, in contrast to Structure A, we work down the quadriceps in order to allow the anterior superior pelvis to drop forward. Our work on the belly and chest is up, as in Structure A.

The legs as shown in Structure A and B are different. In A there is excessive plantar-flexion (with the heel lifting and the weight going forward onto the ball of the foot), so the arrow for our stroke is downward. But in Structure B the weight is more on the heels and there is excess dorsi flexion in front. (The toes may be somewhat drawn up). Now the directions are up in back and down in the front.

In the case of all these strokes you can move longitudinally along the muscle and at the same time gradually hook diagonally across the myofascial structure.

3. Use these two handed strokes across major joints with interacting movements. For example, working on the medial knee, one hand will be moving down along the upper medial calf, while the other will be moving up along the vastus lateralis. Here the work is across the joint, but still respects the principle of working down on the back of the body and up on the front (the medial calf is posterior to the tibia; the vastus lateralis is anterior to the gracilis).

166

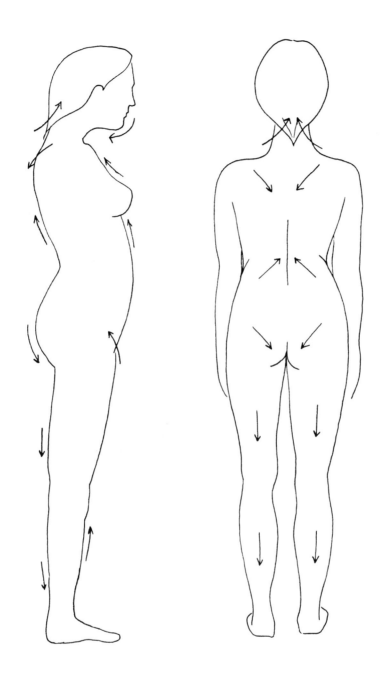

DIRECTION OF MOVEMENT OF BODY SEGMENTS STRUCTURE A

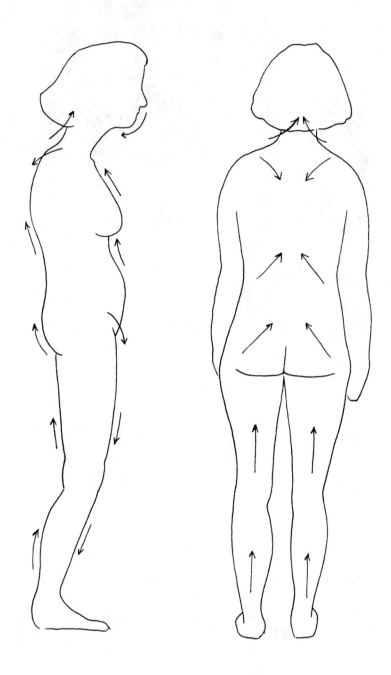

DIRECTION OF MOVEMENT OF BODY SEGMENTS STRUCTURE B

4. Do not overwork the halves of the body. We are now concerned with integration. If we work both on the agonists and antagonists of an imbalance, we will simply reinforce the imbalance.

BREATH AND ENERGY WORK

By this phase of the work, the cycle of charge and discharge should be more even than in the beginning sessions. Work now on sustaining the charge and sustaining the discharge. There should be less hyperventilation and its attendant tetany. There is more consciousness of being in control of one's energy. Explore how it's possible to breath fast, without overexerting oneself, or how it's possible to breathe deeply without trying. Use the "sustained" and "connected" breath frequently.

MOVEMENT AWARENESS

Try out movements which involve the whole body. For example, while the client is on the back with knees bent, the knees are moved by moving the feet up at the ankle. Simultaneously, the pelvis is curled with the psoas (extrinsics remain relaxed) during an inhalation. Also during the inhalation, the chin drops to meet the rising chest. During the exhalation the pelvis, feet drop and the chin lifts slightly. These movements can be used as a total body interaction of the client with your organizing strokes. You can add to the movement a pulling down of the elbows (during inhalation), while the shoulders remain stabilized by the rhomboids in back. These movements should be "empty," zen-like images which are not goals, but merely pictures which one does not try to execute.

MERIDIANS AND POINTS

1. Use mostly Self Regulating points, Doors of life and Windows to the sky. There should be less need for stimulation or sedation.

2. Brush the full length of meridians. Be sure to brush both the yin and yang groups, preferably simultaneously.

CHAKRAS

1. As in the last phase, use mudras which allow you to move along all the chakras. Remember that in some meditations the movement of energy is not just from the basal chakra up through the head chakra, but also down from the head to the bottom. Kundalini uncoils but can also recoil.

2. Tantric closing of the gates (closing all the orifices, and entering an internal state), can help unify bodymind. Also using CV1 along with the third eye or GV1 with GV16 helps connect energies.

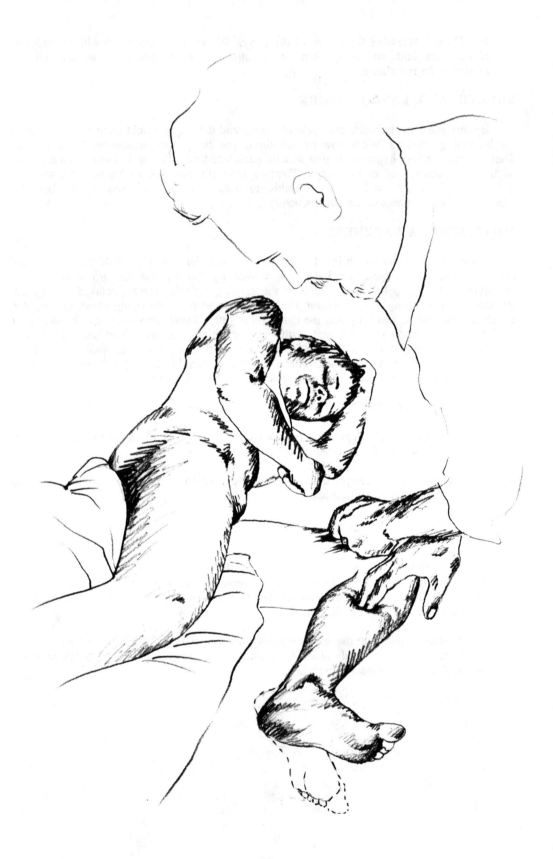

SESSION 8 AND 9

(Upper and Lower Halves)

CHOOSING BETWEEN TWO HALVES

The assumption in beginning this phase of the work is that the first seven sessions have been effective. If there is still major armor in some parts of bodymind, it may be necessary to return to an earlier point in the process. You may need to redo the seventh session, or even return to the fourth session. In any case, continue the sequence from the point where you re-begin, (i.e., after session 4, do 5, 6, and 7, before trying to complete the last phase). If the sequence has been effective, there will be a noticeable change in the quality of the tissue. The layers of tissue will now be even in the distribution of their tension. There will be an equal responsiveness from the superficial down to the deep layers.

The two horizontal halves of our body are often very different. The upper half may be expanded and developed, while the lower half may be smaller and less developed. Or just the opposite may be the case: the upper half thin, small, maybe even collapsed; the lower broad, fleshy, and strong. This contrast is not merely a physical phenomenon, for our whole character is involved. When we use one half of ourselves to manipulate the other half, as well as other people, we develop these top-heavy or bottom-heavy disproportions. As top-heavy we may be socially manipulative, but ungrounded. As bottom heavy we may be seductive, but socially insecure.

By the integrative stage these two halves are free of much of their armor, but need to be coordinated with each other. When working with one half of bodymind, the practitioner needs to encourage movement, energy, and consciousness in the other half. Picture the body as an unopened flower bud. After the first stage of release, the petals are looser and ready to open, but either the lower or upper parts of the petals are more stuck. One strategy for starting the connecting or opening process is to work in one session on the half which is least ready to open, that is, the half which still has comparatively more myofascial disorganization and restriction, as well as less emotional and mental consciousness. The freeing of this half of the body affects the other end of the petals in the other half as well.

In the accompanying diagram, the top heavy man provides an illustration of how his smaller, underdeveloped lower half needs to be opened first. The bottom heavy woman provides an illustration of how her small, tight upper part needs to be opened first. I usually begin sessions 8 and 9 in the middle of the body at the level of the waist. If I have chosen to work on the lower half, I work downward into the remaining deep tensions of the pelvis and legs and thereby free fascial planes which allow the thoracic cage (upper half) to begin to lift out of the pelvis (lower half). Loosening the lower half helps unfold the upper half, and the opening process is then continued in the next session, 9, by working directly with the upper half.

But if the top of the flower bud is tighter -- that is if the diaphragm, back, chest, or neck is still too contracted at the level of the deepest layers of fascia -- I again start at the waist but begin releasing the petals in the top half. In the next session I can then work with the bottom half. We can change the metaphor for a moment to an image of the last chapter: the rib cage floating like a parachute above, while the pelvis and legs dangle below. In the illustration you can see the chest being lifted by the broad distribution of body weight and tension in the upper half of the body. This happens when the myofascial network of tissue is evenly distributed around the whole rib cage, taking pressure away from individual ribs or vertebrae. This even expansion above, in turn, promotes a descending flexibility in breathing and movement down through the belly, hips, sacrum, and legs. It is worth noting that the bones are not the major support in an integrated body; but rather it is the fascia, when properly organized, which really bears the body weight. When the fascia is free, the bones move easily in fine, crisp articulations with each other.

171

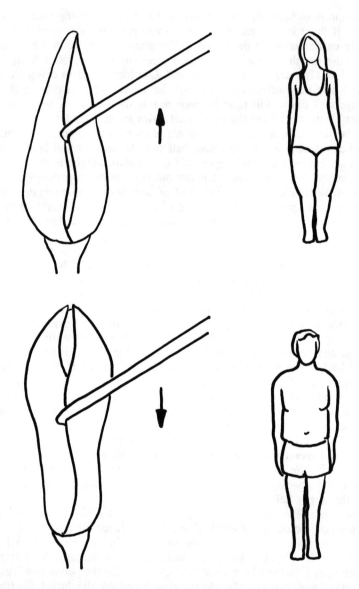

When the process of deep bodywork has reached the stage of integration -- sessions 8, 9, 10 -- the body can be likened to a flower bud whose petals are ready to open from the middle. If the top is still relatively tight, the petals are first opened upward in session 8. The next session, 9, then completes the opening. Session 10 encourages a harmonious balance throughout the whole, now completely open, structure.

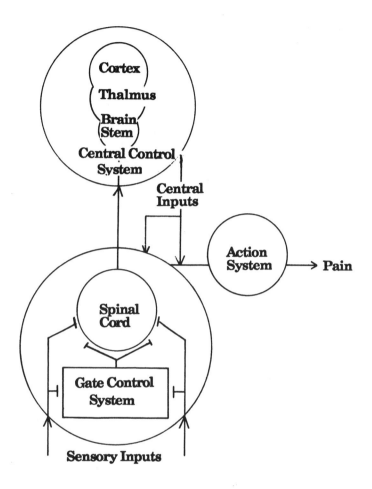

According to one of the classical explanations, pain is a conditioned response in the brain to a simple outside stimulus to the tissue. But this view does not account for the contribution which local tissue makes to the experience of pain. What we experience as pain depends on how local tissue allows the stimulus to be received; it depends on the "memory" held in the tissues. Here we see an alternative to the classical model. The nervous system is a reciprocal unit, such that changes in any one part affect every other part. The nervous system uses a complicated set of gates which open and close as stimuli pass through local receptors.

A TEST FOR KNOWING WHICH HALF IS FIRST

If it is not visually clear which half you should work with, try the following test. Begin working at the middle of the body (lateral gluteals) and work either downward or upward in the direction you feel might be appropriate. After a few minutes of work, the release of tissue where you are working should have produced an expanding, rocking release in the movement of the breathing in the other half, on which you have not worked, either a breath upward into the cage --if you have chosen to work on the lower half-- or a breath downward into the sacrum and buttocks, if you have chosen to work on the upper half.

COMBINING THE TWO HALVES

But it is not always the case that we are either more closed on the top or on the bottom. It may be the case that your model is partly open, and partly closed on the top -- or the same may be true on the bottom half. It is possible to modify our strategy, beginning at the middle, but working in the eighth session part of the way toward the top, and part of the way toward the bottom, and in the 9th session finishing the work on both halves.

BODYREADING

1.   Consider top or bottom heavy, or combined characteristics as discussed above. Help your model get in touch with these parts of themselves.

2.   Begin looking at the long lines of the body. See how hip, knee, and ankle can function better along a straight line; how the hip, shoulder and neck work together; how the tension shifts from side to side or from front to back, etc.

3.   Develop a strategy, realizing that you may have to change the strategy as you go along. You will need to look at your client in a standing position, frequently throughout the session.

BODY AREAS (for the bottom half)

1.   **Middle of the Body**. Begin around the gluteals, abductors, adductors, iliacus, and psoas. This part of the body has so many layers of tissue, so many connections in all directions that it is a major unravelling and release point for bodymind. Work toward the extremities, that is, first around the pelvis, the upper legs, then around the lower legs, etc.

2.   **Abduction and Adduction**. Work toward alignment of the leg. Perhaps one hip will need to have its abduction lessened, while the other will need its adduction lessened. But somewhere on the same leg, the tension and disorganization will shift to the other side. If you work on the gluteus minimus and medialis, somewhere along the same leg, perhaps in the lower leg, there will be a counter pull (tibialis posterior). On the other leg their may also be a shifting of tension, but an opposite pattern: from the adductors in the upper leg to the peroneals in the lateral lower leg.

BODY READING: See what's happening.

3.   **Intrinsics of the Pelvis**. Before working on the lower legs, return to the pelvis (principle of working from the middle toward the extremities). Pay particular attention to balancing the iliopsoas and the deep lateral rotators in the buttocks. Work on the attachments.

A. Work with the fingers of one hand, along the medial surface of the ischium, interacting with the obturator internus, while working with the other hand on   the

174

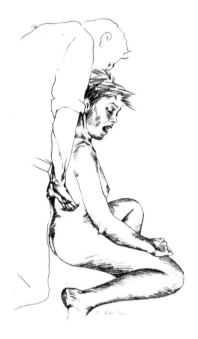

Release of shortened and thickened fascia covering the back of the waist line (quadratus lmborum) helps in lengthening, balancing and increasing the mobility of the middle of the body.

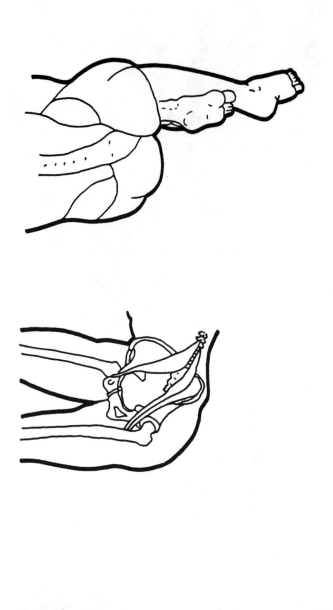

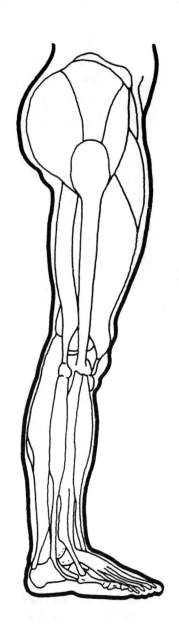

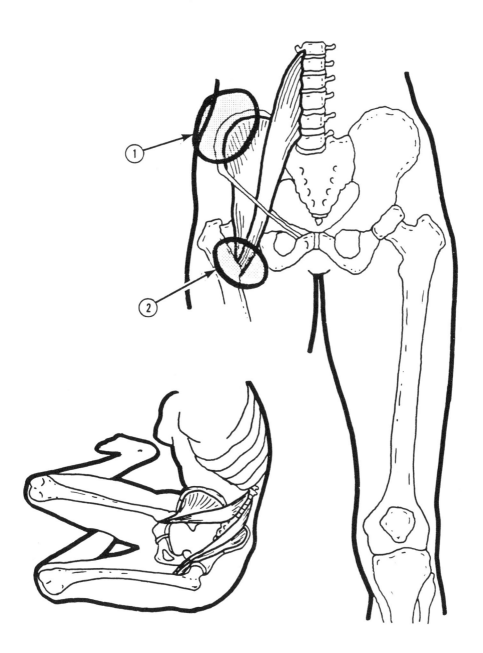

body of the psoas. A rocking motion of the pelvis, with external rotation, will help with the interaction.

B. Iliacus. From a sidesaddle position, reach inside the higher hip with both fingertips. Slowly penetrate deep into the iliacus, while the client rocks the pelvis. This not only releases contractions which pull downward in the iliopsoas, but also encourages elongation of the side of the body, a lifting of the cage out of the pelvis.

C. Try working on the sacrum, while your model is lying over the edge of the table, knees on the floor, belly on the table top. It is important that the knees be elevated to a proper height. Also use a pillow or table foam to protect that part of the front of the pelvis pushing against the table. Use elbows strokes (down and in toward the mid line) to organize the sacral tissue. Model rocks the pelvis.

BODY READING: Look again.

4. **Knees.**

A. When the entire knee is turned inward, look at the function of the popliteus (inward rotation of the tibialis), at the tension on the medial knee (gracilis, vastus medialis), and in some cases at the peroneals (collapse of the inner arch by overcontraction of lateral foot).

B. When the entire knee is turned out, look at the contraction in the vastus lateralis and sartorius (rotates and flexes the knee).

C. Since the knee is the meeting of the femur, tibia and fibula, there can be a twisting at the knee, with part of the leg (and knee) turning in, and part turning out.

D. Locked knees. Work to loosen the quadriceps by working on the attachments at both ends of these muscles.

E. Flexed knees. In a few rare cases the knees are bent too far. Look for a shortened hamstrings.

BODY READING: Stand your client up again.

5. **Ankles and Arches.** Look at the horizontal axis passing through the two malleoli. Looking at how this line is tilted to one side or the other as well as toward the back or front, can help you see the stress in the foot. The weight of the foot should be evenly distributed along three arches:

A. Lateral arch. When this arch is flat, the lateral peroneal muscles are overworking, and the medial supporters of the arch are weak. The adductors (gracilis) may also be stuck, preventing the lower medial muscles from contracting. Work along the fibula, which may be rotated forward, and with the adductors of the thigh.

B. Medial arch. This arch may become overly developed as compensation for a weak lateral arch. You may also find tension underneath in the lateral plantar region.

C. Transverse arch. When the instep is high and narrow, work not only to flatten it, by working directly on it from above, but also work with the medial plantar fascia underneath. On top the tibialis anterior and the peroneus tertius may also be involved.

D. Notice that while the medial arch on one foot is collapsed, the medial arch on the other foot is overdeveloped. This may be part of a pattern which is seen as abduction of one thigh and adduction of the other, or elevation of one shoulder and depression of the other.

6. Pelvic curl, neck, and back. Usual strokes.

FINAL BODY READING AND FINE ENERGY

Spend plenty of time helping your client feel the new directions of body organization. Alexander images, and Feldenkrais explorations are helpful. Use the above mentioned affirmations along with the body movements. Use Windows to the Sky and other points to lift energy after having worked on the lower half. Notice how the upper half of the body is lifting out of the lower half, although you have not worked on the upper half.

BODY AREA (upper half)

Allow enough time to pass (two weeks minimum) for the body to begin to find a new direction, for the changes to be assimilated. An exception: if a person is very unstable and has a tendency to easily fall back into a disorganized state. In this case it might be good to do 8 and 9 a few days apart, fitting one half of the body on the other, then wait a few weeks for session 10.

1. Lateral Torso. Begin at gluteals and work up along the side of the body, as in the beginning of session 3. Use cross-handed strokes to connect the torso and pelvis. On one side, the quadratus lumborum may be more contracted than on the other. It may not be necessary to work both sides. But do not work all the way to the shoulder, before you have returned to other parts of the pelvis. Work a little on each side, as you work toward the extremities.

BODY READING. Stand your client up and share the results.

2. Abdominus Rectus. Rework attachments, beginning at pubis. Work upward in zigzags, then do attachments on the ribs.

3. Diaphragm. Try to reach the attachments. Give plenty of support on the inside of the ribs with the other hand. If you have any difficulty getting into the diaphragm, rework the psoas with both hands. Reach toward its origins, high on the lumbar spine. This will help release the diaphragm, as well as the dorsal spine.

BODY READING: Observe.

4. Rhomboids. While the client is sitting, work on the rhomboids and anterior cage simultaneously. The shoulders need to be anchored, the arms moving slightly, and the inhalation full. Pull down in the back with one hand and lift in the front with the other.

BODY READING: Again, observe.

5. Arms. Notice the rotation of the arms and consider whether to focus on lateral or medial rotation, and work under the arm or on the shoulder blade. Also look at whether the arm is chronically flexed at the elbow. Work deep on the attachments of the biceps. Or if there is hyperextension, on the triceps at the elbow. It is important to

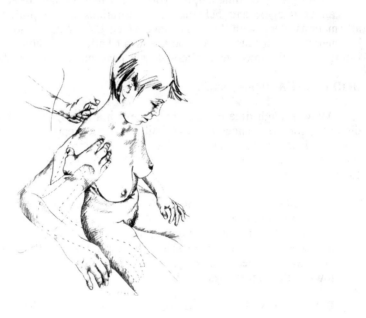

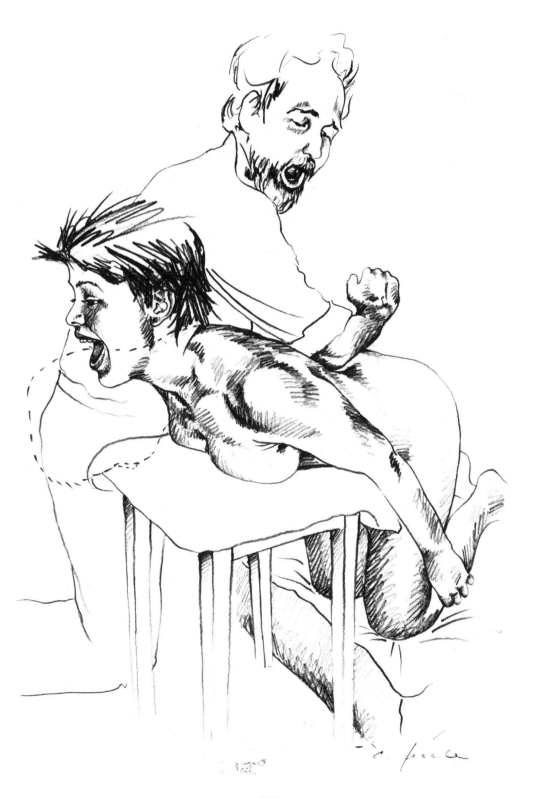

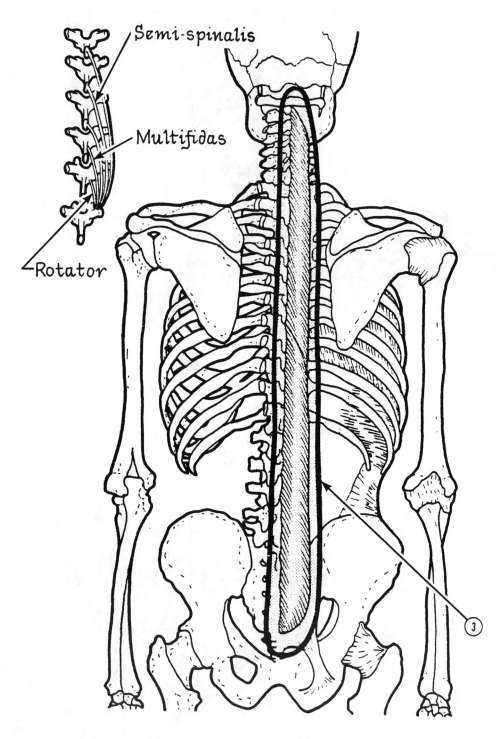

Semi-spinalis

Multifidas

Rotator

3

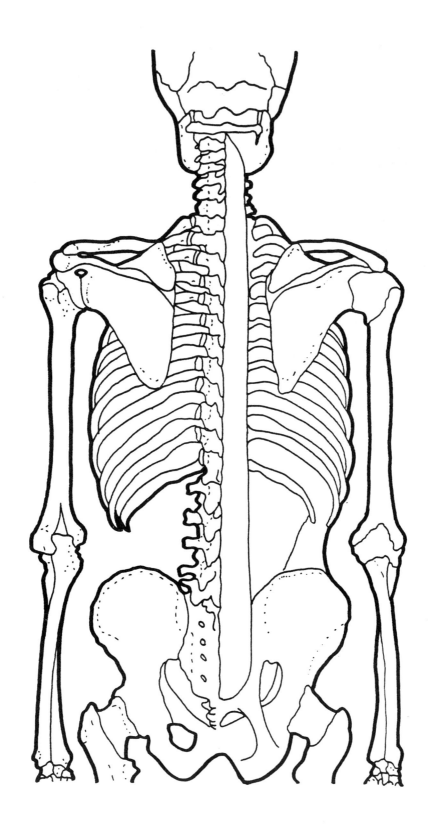

connect and coordinate the space between the insertion of the triceps and the mid-thoracic area. There needs to be enough distance for the elbow to move forward, while the shoulder stays anchored by the rhomboids and pectoralis minor. Also notice that the forward position of the arm is not always caused by the shoulder (pectoralis major) but may involve excessive pronation of the forearm. Go to the attachments of the pronators. Check out supination as well.

6.   Subscapularis. Perhaps during the third session you were not able to reach very far under the shoulder blade in trying to contact the subscapularis. Now it should be much more available. Be sure your model is aware of how to control the position of the shoulders, while the arms move up and down and are rotated.

BODYREADING: Again share with your model.

7.   Shoulder. When the pectoralis minor is overcontracted, you may need to work both the origin and insertion. Notice that this is often needed on only one side. When working on the top of the shoulder (supraspinatus, trapezius, levator scapula), be sure the shoulders are anchored, and that there is awareness of the distance between the shoulder tips and the ears. Rotation of the head on a perpendicular axis through the neck can help with the reorganization of the shoulders. When the shoulders are elevated, work along the top and medial upper border of the shoulder blades. You will be cutting across the levator scapula and some fibers of the trapezius. Be sure your client remains straight, not tilting one shoulder down as you work. You may have to stand on the table and support your client's torso with your knee. Also during your stroke the shoulder blades remain stable and the client explores movements with the arm and neck (chin is dropped). This is similar to work in session 3.

BODY READING: Stand client up.

8.   Neck and Mouth. If the neck is still too far forward, now is the time to again work at the attachments of the sternocleidomastoid and inside the mouth on the tongue. Also the attachment of the capitis muscles, along the occiput, can be very important.

9.   Sacral Curl, Neck, And Back.   Usual strokes.

FINAL BODY READING AND FINE ENERGY

As in the last session, use movement awareness and affirmations together.   Use grounding points after having worked on the upper half.   Notice how breathing descends toward the knees although you have not worked on the lower half.

SESSION 10

(Fine Tuning the Whole Structure)

The final session begins at the feet and continues to the head. It is a very selective session. Do not overwork the structure. Give a minimal number of directions for change and let the individual find his or her own integration, over a period of weeks or months. Studying several possible types of structural patterns will help organize your strategies.

1. **Left-right.** Example: the tension shifts from one side of the body to the other; one ankle is collapsed; the opposite hip is too high; the other shoulder down and forward.

2. **Front-back.** Tension in the achilles tendon shifts forward into locked knees; this shifts into a swayed back; again forward to the diaphragm; into the upper shoulder blades. Or in another case the tension is in the tibialis anterior and shifts to the hamstrings.

3. **Inside-outside.** Flat feet (outside tension) go to knock knees (inside), to short waist (outside), to pinched diaphragm (inside), to shoulders forward (outside). Or high arches (tension inside) to abducted hips (outside), to diaphragm (inside), to shoulders outside.

4. **Repeating.** The tension in the ankles can be seen again in the belly, again in the throat.

5. **Twisting.** When one knee is bent more than the other, this difference is part of an unequal contraction in the iliopsoas and obliques, and can be seen in a twisted neck and head.

BODY AREAS

In following these patterns of tension. it is not necessarily the case that you will want to work directly on the line of tension which you have traced from one part of the body to another. The lines of tension show where a change is needed, but you may need to work at some distance from this line of tension. For example, if the tension of knock-knee-legs moves upward from the outer ankles toward the inner knee, you may not wish to do most of your work around the knees. It may be more important to work on the upper attachments of the adductors at the pubis (gracilis, pectineus, adductor brevis). These lines of tension are merely reference points which show where the imbalance makes itself evident, but the problem probably begins in the disorganization of tissue some distance from this point. Also when following a pattern, you may not need to work every part of the pattern. In the case of a tight diaphragm, which is part of a pattern with bow legs, you might work only on the legs and not directly touch the diaphragm, although you would be judging the effectiveness of your work by degree of opening you are able to achieve in the diaphragm. Use the principle: "Work where the symptom isn't."

FINAL BODY READING AND FINE ENERGY

Look at the "before session 1" and "after session 10" photographs. It is important that you point out the details of the changes. It is very difficult for clients to look objectively at themselves. Also point out that without any further work there will be many changes in the following months. Often there are more changes after, than during the process. Point out the areas that need more awareness and tailor a few exercises to fit these problems; run through them at least once with your client. If the client is interested in more sessions, but has already reached a saturation point, suggest a self-integrating period of a few months, before another session 10 (or advanced work, if you are qualified). Point out that if a stressful environment hasn't been changed, that one may be more aware of the stress, and less likely to tolerate it. Once the body has been released and reorganized, it is, of course, possible to accumulate tension and to lose part of one's balance, but emphasize that bodymind also has a greater capacity to re-release and reorganize itself. Often, simply letting go of feelings and going through some movement awareness exercises is enough to bring one back to a fine balance.

One important affirmation is to work with the feelings and idea of completion. Often we burden ourselves with the idea that we never finish with our problems. If we stay with the here and now it is possible to say, "I'm complete; I'm finished." The fact that in the next moment we have different feelings need not take away from the completeness of the present moment. Have your model explore the feeling of being finished.

BODYWORK JOURNAL

Curtiss Turchin and Jack Painter

BEFORE SESSION 1

Try to skip two meals before your sessions. If this is difficult, skip a minimum of one meal. It is recommended that fresh juice and tea be substituted for these two meals. Camomille, mint and comfrey tea are especially good, as they are natural calmatives and healing teas. It is not recommended that you drink coffee or take drugs of any kind before a session. The wrong kind of substance in your system can increase the likelihood of discomfort and can diminish the results.

Vitamin C and E speeds healing of tissue, and calcium helps the tissue relax. Some evidence suggests that the Bioflavonoids can help diminished bruising. Try these supplements before and in between each session.

Give yourself the space to have a free, quiet evening after the session. The experience of Postural Integration is deep and emotional, and in order to learn as much as possible, give yourself a chance to feel quiet and separate from the rest of your hectic life.

A good follow-up to this work is a sauna or hot tub. If these facilities are unavailable to you, a hot bath with oil and/or herbs is a soothing way of mellowing out after the experience of a session.

It is expected that "unfinished business" will surface for you for days, even weeks after a session. Let these feelings surface so that you may observe your deeper, less conscious levels. Let your friends know that you will be in a very emotional space for a while. Be specific in asking them to support you in this experience.

If you have anything specific with which you want to work -- diet, emotional problems, physical pains -- let your practitioner know before the session begins. Within the process of Postural Integration there are specific areas and strategies which will receive attention. Yet, each session is to be tailored to your individual needs. Don't be afraid to ask for help.

Draw a picture of yourself with colored crayons showing your body image, color of your aura and posture. Doing this after each session is a good way to focus on where you are and how you have changed.

SESSION 1

DISCUSSION

Session one begins to unravel the blocked tissue around the chest and diaphragm. There is a strong emphasis during the session on freeing your breathing. A fuller, freer breath will improve your circulation and consequently improve the oxygenation of all tissues and cells. Opening your chest and diaphragm will also allow your feelings to surface more easily.

This session can reawaken you and give you a new enthusiasm for life. Welcome this feeling of freshness and inspiration. Realize too that the unrealistic fantasies you harbor will become clearer to you. Look at what you have invested in them and feel the sadness that comes from their emptiness.

QUESTIONS

1. What feelings surfaced which you worked on or expressed?
2. What feelings were not expressed?
3. Notice that you do not allow some feelings to come out.
4. What feelings are in your chest? Do you often feel like you need to get things off your chest?
5. Do you let it be o.k. for you to get excited?

EXERCISE

While lying on your back or standing, place a hand on each side of your ribs and concentrate on expanding in every direction around your cage and diaphragm. Surrender to a full inhalation and exhalation without forcing either.

SESSION 2

DISCUSSION

Sessions one and two are on a layer of superficial tissue which lies just beneath the skin. This layer is like a large shopping bag which organizes the entire body contents. If we have made this outside layer hard and protective, the tissue work during these first sessions may at times be painful. This is often the case for session two, since it covers the legs where we store all of our concerns about our grounding, all our insecurity about standing on our own two feet.

Pain is not always an indication that we have to tighten our bodies and defend ourselves. Often if we relax into pain and allow ourselves to fully experience it, it changes into a feeling of relief or release, or an emotion which we have been hiding may have a chance to come to consciousness and be dealt with.

It is common for this work to bring up past feelings of hurt. The brain is not our only storehouse of memories. The entire nervous system, including brain, spinal cord, spinal nerves and all other nervous tissues help store our experiences. Deep work where we are holding these memories, can help us relive them and more fully claim them as a part of ourselves.

Remember that when deep bodywork is being done, relaxation and deep breathing help to reduce the intensity of pain and trauma. Deep breathing helps build a high level of charging and discharging energy which, in turn, helps promote a permanent reorganization of the tissues being released.

QUESTIONS

1. Did you find this session painful?
2. What parts of your body did you tighten in response to pain?
3. Where do you protect yourself?
4. How did you deal with discomfort and pain as a child? Have you changed? What is the difference?
5. Do you deal with physical and emotional pain in the same way?

EXERCISE

Spend a few minutes each day massaging your feet. After you soften them, notice how they make better contact with the earth.

SESSION 3

DISCUSSION

Session three will help you feel longer along the sides of your body and free the upper part of your arms so that you are better in touch with the feeling of reaching out and holding back.

Notice that we are often short in the waist and stiff when we try to bend from side to side. As part of this shortness and stiffness there is often a flattening and swaying of back. By lengthening ourselves, we become more flowing and sensual, and we allow ourselves to become rounder and straighter.

Notice that arms sometimes turn in and the shoulders come forward, or they may turn out, while the shoulders are pulled back, exposing the chest. Often we do not want to use our arms to express our needs. We are reaching but never receiving; we are holding back, even as we bravely "take it on the chest." Deep work under the arms helps us contact and release these chronically held attitudes.

QUESTIONS

1. Are you short or stiff along the sides of your torso?
2. Are you afraid to let your body flow in sensual movements from side to side?
3. How do you hold your arms and shoulders?
4. Do you hesitate to reach out to people, to embrace them? 5. Did you hug your mom and dad as you were growing up?

EXERCISE

Lie on your back with your knees bent. As you exhale reach up with your arms and shoulders, letting your head fall back and your knees fall apart. As you inhale return your arms and shoulders and bring your knees together. With each exhalation go further into what you feel. Try crying out for help. Call for "mommy" and "daddy." Try "I want you," or "I need you."

SESSION 4

DISCUSSION

In sessions three we reached a level physically and emotionally deeper than in sessions one or two. Now in session four we are beginning to touch the core of your bodymind. It is important that at this point you have a full commitment to the Postural Integration process. Fundamental changes will begin which need to be completed. If you stop, you may be confused and frustrated.

We will be working with the quadriceps and adductors of the thighs. The quadriceps often are chronically stiff from our attempts to hold our knees rigid, to make sure everything stays secure. The adductors may be squeezing our legs together to protect the groin.

During this session let the anger, fear and frustration which you have locked in the pelvis be expressed through your belly, chest and throat. Your practitioner may from time to time help you with the gag reflex and may encourage you to yell or cry.

QUESTIONS

1. Do you bend your knees when standing normally?
2. Are you willing to surrender, to be a little weak in the knees?
3. Do you hold your legs close together?
4. Do you feel comfortable opening your legs, exposing your genitals?
5. Can you feel your legs separate from your pelvis, forming round, supporting columns?

EXERCISES

1. Balance yourself on one leg and bend your knee, gradually going toward the floor. At some point let yourself fall forward or backward, giving a yell. The point of this exercise is to let yourself surrender. Try falling forward or backward onto a mattress.

2. Lie on your back with your knees bent and spread apart. Grab the gracilis (large tendon attaching to the pubis inside the thighs) with both hands. Massage deeply, breathing deeply and expressing the pleasure, fear, or pain locked inside your legs.

SESSION 5

DISCUSSION

This session will help you examine the relationship between your "core" and your "shell." Your core is your "being" and your shell is your "doing." Your core is your spontaneity, effortlessness, withdrawal, or your place inside. The muscles of the internal organs, the bones, and the intrinsic muscles help to initiate and coordinate the large movements which are powered by our outer muscles. The "shell" is concerned with business, taking action, and carrying out plans. It is the reflection of our will and desire to accomplish things. It has to do with attitudes, postures, and roles. The "shell" is generally composed of the large extrinsic musculature of the arms, legs and back. Shell personalities often lack grace in movement because they use their muscles to "keep it all together." Lacking inner directed movement, they often appear jerky and strained when they move. These persons are often muscle-bound or the last one to pick up the steps in a social dance class. The core personality has an easy time moving in slow subtle movements. Yet, their lack of a strong external musculature does not permit them the opportunity for full, expressive movement. Core personalities may not show their anger for fear of being "out there," where they might need a shield for their flaccid musculature. One of the main goals of the PI process is to unify our inner and outer actions, to help us discover both our outer and inner selves.

The psoas is an important intrinsic muscle, lying deep in the pelvis. The practitioner will help you to begin initiating pelvic movements from this inner muscle, rather than from the belly and buttocks.

Also this session, which covers the chest, belly, and front of the pelvis, can help you connect your pelvis and chest, your sexuality and heart feelings.

QUESTIONS

1. Are you more of a core or shell personality?
2. When do you use your core and when do you use your shell?
3. Are you able to move between these two spaces?
4. When is your shell hardest? When is your core softest?
5. Are your relationships sometimes either sexual without deep feelings, or friendly without sensuality?
6. Can you accept both excitement and closeness?

EXERCISE

While lying on your back with the knees bent, slightly curl your pelvis upward toward your chin, without tightening your belly or buttocks. Breath deeply and softly. While you breathe rapidly, pant and rock your pelvis. Hold one hand on your genitals, the other over your heart.

SESSION 6

DISCUSSION

This session will help you feel the connection between the back of your pelvis and your legs. The rotators (deep butt muscles) have the ability to rotate the legs in and out. Some authorities say that the feet should be optimally parallel when at rest. This places the feet slightly apart and straight ahead. Others say that a slight outward turn is necessary for most efficient movement. Generally, it is agreed that feet pointing too far outward puts strain on the ankles, knees, and hips. Charlie Chaplin's grossly exaggerated outward turn of the feet make him comical, weak, and uncoordinated. Your feet and legs determine your relationship to the earth.

When the rotators are chronically overcontracted this tension is part of a pattern of anal holding back. Here we find deep anger against mommy and daddy, who forced us to control our shit. This may be anger against any kind of authority. When we let go of this held back rage, we can again feel relief and pleasure.

QUESTIONS

1. Do your feet, legs, and hips feel comfortable when properly aligned?
2. Have you ever met someone and experienced a "pain in the ass." Imagine this person in front of you, and try expressing your anger.
3. When you feel weak or guilty, do you tuck your tail under?
4. Do you stick your rear out in the air, hiding your genitals, but inviting someone to kick you in the ass.
5. Is it o.k. to rub your anus? Is this pleasant?

EXERCISE

Stand in your normal posture. Now, turn your feet out as far as they will move to the side -- experience this. Turn your feet inward until you are slightly pigeon toed -- experience this. Find a position in between these two -- experience this. With your feet in this optimal alignment, unlock your knees, being conscious of maintaining feet and knees pointing forward.

SESSION 7

DISCUSSION

Matthias Alexander calls the head the "primary control center." This means that the head is the leader of all movement. When we move forward, the head leads the way. If there is tension in the back of the neck, we will, when we stand or sit, tend to arch the neck backward. Even when we are standing still and under a great deal of stress, the head will often jut forward. When our heads are out of alignment there are always corresponding tensions in the rest of the body. A well aligned head and neck will help bring the rest of the body into proper alignment from shoulders to toes!

Not only is the head a leader in the physical use of the body, but it also is the "governor of expression." As the governor of expression, it only allows us to smile, laugh, cry, etc. when the throat and facial channels are open. Pursing the lips holds back the whimper; clenching the teeth restricts the scream; and clamping down on the tongue prohibits the smile. Deep connective tissue work on the head and neck region helps us to move our faces in ways we have forgotten and thought impossible. Rather than restricting us, the head can then be a vehicle of our true feelings. After this session many people feel they have taken off their masks.

QUESTIONS

1. What emotion is most difficult for you to express? What part of your face blocks its expression?
2. What scares you about having your mouth and nose intruded upon?
3. What is happening when you feel your face like a mask?
4. What do you like about your face?
5. What do you dislike about it?

EXERCISE

Look at yourself very closely in the mirror every day. Get in touch with what pleases and displeases you. Make many faces -- horror, anger, grief, outrage, etc. Exaggerate those expressions which are most difficult for you.

SESSIONS 8, 9, 10

DISCUSSION

Sessions 8, 9, and 10 will give you an opportunity to learn new relationships with gravity. Sessions 8 and 9 will deal with either the top or bottom half of the body. Session 10 will integrate the whole body.

Posture is the way we choose to relate to gravity. As our posture begins to improve our body experiences profound psychological and physiological changes. Bodymind now begins to vibrate all over. When we breathe, move or feel, the body responds with "streaming" energy. Tensions and different emotions move through us more easily. We begin to have a feeling of unity, of wholeness.

Consider yourself from different perspectives -- mentally, spiritually, emotionally, and physically. Notice changes in your life during Postural Integration. Where do you feel you need to go from here?

This series of ten sessions is meant to help you through major changes in your life. If you feel the need to do more work, there are sequels to the ten sessions which can make the process even more complete.

QUESTIONS

1. Of which half of you are you more conscious, the lower or upper half?
2. How does one half give support to the other half? Create a dialogue between the two halves.
3. When you inhale, how far can you feel the breath travel up and down your body. To the top of your head? All the way down to your feet?

EXERCISES

1. Close your eyes and allow your conscious mind to be a bright, colored liquid which radiates downward and outward from your brain to fill your whole body with light. Feel the color in your toes.

2. Imagine your body to be composed of blocks which may be shifted at will to become more stable. Your blocks are head, shoulders, chest, belly, pelvis, knees and feet. 3. Sit in a comfortable chair with your feet firmly on the ground and your knees even with your hip sockets. Imagine head, shoulders, chest, stomach, and pelvic blocks to be brightly colored. The rest of your body is black. Begin to gently shift your body blocks until you feel each block stacked to obtain the maximum straightness without any tension. If you feel tight, repeat the process until you can align these blocks and still be comfortable.

INDEX

TRAINING CENTERS IN ENGLISH SPEAKING COUNTRIES

UNITED STATES

The International Center for Release and Integration is located near San Francisco (mailing address: Jack Painter, 450 Hillside Avenue, Mill Valley, CA 94941; Tel. 415-383-4017). Information about training programs and certified practitioners is available. The following centers also give trainings and can recommend practitioners.

LOS ANGELES
Jack Haer and Mary Treiger, Bodymind Institute, 11081 Missouri Avenue, L.A., CA 90025, Tel. 213-473-5737.

FLORIDA
Joyce Johnson, Florida Institute of Psychophysical Integration, 5837 Mariner Drive, Tampa, FL 33609, Tel. 813-877-2273.

COLORADO
Billy Gunter, Quantum Leap Enterprises, 1015 11th Street, Boulder, CO 80302, Tel. 303-442-1952.

MISSOURI
Nirmal Karros, 2101 Arsenal, St. Louis, MO 63118, Tel. 314-772-8848.

HAWAII
Shawn Thompson and Kathy Boyles, 126 Onekea Dr., Kailua, HI 96734, Tel. 808-261-0433.

Kathy and Don Hallock, 3101 Huelani Pl., Honolulu, HI 96822, Tel. 808-988-4874.

NEW YORK
Susanne Gruber, 1594 Third Avenue, New York, NY 10028, Tel. 212-289-2405.

Norman Early, 432 Winter Street, Troy, NY 12180.

NEW JERSEY
Barron Dixon, 388 Ramapo Valley Rd., Oakland, NJ 07436, Tel. 201-337-9242.

CANADA
(English and French)

Jean Pierre Chartrand, 3950 Drolet St., Montreal H2W 2L2, Tel. 514-844-0751.

ENGLAND

Silke Ziehl, 14 Glamorgan Rd., Hampton Wick, Kingston Upon Thames, Surrey KT1 4HP, Tel. 019772226.

Freda Copley, 2 Woodvale Terr Hawksworth Rd., Horsforth, Leeds, Tel. 8945228.

Sean Doherty, 465 Queen's Rd., Sheffield S240R, Tel (0742) 558165.

Susan Sidery, Old Scholhouse, Dunkeswell Abbey, Honiton, Devon (Hemycock), Tel. 680537.

SCOTLAND

Ian Holland, 128 Byres Rd., Hillhead, Glasgow, Tel. 0413345846.

Robert Anderson, 29 Lawnston Place, Edinburgh, EH3909. Tel. (301) 2281183.

AUSTRALIA

Deva Daricha, Greenwood Lane Centre, Box 233, Yarra Glen, Victoria 3775.

CENTERS IN COUNTRIES WITH OTHER LANGUAGES

Contact Mill Valley for centers or practitioners in France, Germany, Sweden, Denmark, Italy, Quebec, Canada, Mexico, Brazil, and Venezuela.

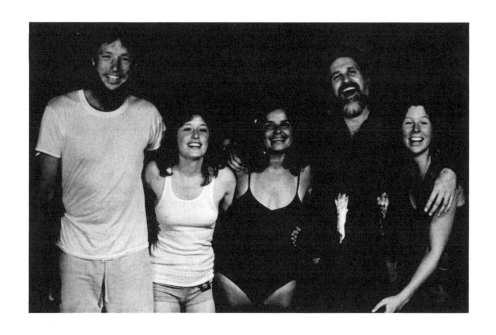

Jack Painter, second from the right, is shown with a group of Postural Integrators. He is director of The International Center for Release and Integration in Mill Valley (near San Francisco) which offers training and certification in Postural Integration, Reichian Release, Rebirthing, and Pelvic-Sexual Release. He received his Ph.D. from Emory University (Atlanta) in 1961. As a Smith-Mundt scholar he pursued post-graduate research in Europe, and while serving as a professor at the University of Miami (1961-69), he also did research in physio-philosophy and psychology -- acupuncture, yoga, zazen, Reichian and Gestalt bodywork, and connective tissue manipulation. He holds a massage therapy degree from Lindsey Hopkins (Miami) and is an associate of the Instituto Wilhelm Reich in Mexico City. Since 1973 he has trained more than 1500 practitiooners of bodywork and has helped establish centers in Europe, Latin America, the U.S., and Canada.

FROM BODYMIND BOOKS

450 Hillside Avenue
Mill Valley, CA 94941
Tel. 415-383-4017

BOOKS

Deep Bodywork and Personal Development, Harmonizing our Bodies, Emotions, and Thoughts. A unique synthesis of deep tissue, gestalt and reichian work. Filled with technique, theory and illustrations. "A major contribution to Western psychology"—Robert Hall, M.D., (Lomi School). "Goes beyond any model I know"—Ron Kurtz (Body Reveals). For general and professional reader.

Birth Is Not Just For Babies, Self-Renewal in Birthing and Parenting. Letting pregnancy, birth and parenting be an opportunity for personal growth. As we parents give birth to and take care of our children, we need to nurture and love ourselves. This is a practical guide to the use of physical, emotional and spiritual energy to uplift and renew the often blocked and drained lives of parents. Publication in the Spring of 1988.

Strong and Soft, Exercises for Both Physical and Emotional Health. Our zealous training of the body can lead not only to uncomfortable tension in the body, but also to emtional rigidity. Even when we try carefully to follow the principles of body balance, our deep inner feelings subtly control and disorganize our movements. Here is a new approach to body building which encourages emotional freedom with overall bodymind strength and balance. Publication in the Autumn of 1987.

NEWSLETTER

Postural Integration New World Newsletter. A bi-yearly publication for practitioners of deep bodywork. It also contains articles of interest for the general reader, e.g., "Pregnancy, Birth and PI", "Facing the Aids Plague With Confidence", $10.00 in U.S. and Canada; $15.00 outside.

VIDEOS

The Power and Joy of Deep Bodywork. A close up view of how deep tissue and breathwork can change our lives. See, first hand, how being deeply touched can open hardened parts of our bodies and release long held-back or suppressed feelings. Includes an explanation, by Jack Painter, of the process of Postural Integration. Color, 30 minutes, release in the Autumn of 1987.

Breath and Life. Our breathing—inhalation and exhalation—is a cycle of charging and discharging energy, which we often cut short. When we do not allow our energy to build completely or to be fully expressed, we create life-long blocks. Through an exploration of the power of breathing, we can open ourselves to excitement, power, softness and love. Follow Jack Painter through many ways of breathing: chest and belly charging, panting, explosive discharging, meditative charging and discharging, and many more. See dramatic, close-up, on-camera changes. Color, 30 minutes, release in the Autumn of 1987.

The Physical Shape of our Thoughts and Feelings. All those unique parts of us—big hips, narrow chests, hunched shoulders—show how our bodies hold everything that has happened to us in life. Our basic feelings and attitudes—neediness, fear, anger, power—are there in the muscles and bones. Jack Painter guides us in seeing this in our own bodies and in other people. For the general viewer. Indispensable for professionals who work with the body and emotions. Color, 30 minutes, release in the Autumn of 1987.

Becoming a Professional in Deep Bodywork. An intimate view of how several students became interested in developing their power to help others, how they struggled with their self-doubts and inner blocks, and how they gained the self confidence and mastery needed for working with clients. Includes scenes of the classroom teaching of Postural Integration, as well as sessions with students working. Color, 30 minutes, release in the Autumn of 1987.

Make checks payable to **"BODYMIND BOOKS"**.